JACK J. GLENWOOD

Solo Fitness: A Guide to Staying Fit Without the Gym Crowd

Discover Effective, Solo Workouts for Those Who Like Privacy and Peace

Contents

Introduction: Embrace the Power of Solo Fitness

I magine this: no waiting for equipment, not feeling rushed, no anxious glances over your shoulder. Just you, your space, and a sense of freedom as you dive into a workout that's all about you—on your terms. For some, the gym is energizing, a place of community and encouragement. But for those of us who crave a solo experience, or just don't feel comfortable in crowds, working out alone unlocks a powerful and personal journey toward fitness, well-being, and self-confidence.

Whether it's the comfort of your living room, a quiet corner of your backyard, or even a park where you can just pop in some earbuds and focus on yourself. Working out alone comes with distinct advantages. Here, we'll uncover why embracing a solo fitness journey is not only effective but can be deeply rewarding. We'll explore the surprising benefits of training without the crowd, how to build confidence from within, and why your personal space might just be the best gym of all.

The Benefits of Working Out Alone

There's something undeniably empowering about working out alone. It's a chance to disconnect from the expectations, pressures, and judgments that sometimes fill a gym and instead reconnect with yourself. When you work out solo, you're free to try new exercises, push your limits, or rest as needed—without worrying about anyone else's schedule or opinions.

In solo fitness, you become your own best coach, I mean who knows you better than you? You can be setting goals that reflect your unique needs. This approach cultivates a deeper understanding of your body, teaching you what works best for you and what doesn't. You'll discover what exercises make you feel strong and energized, and which ones allow you to release stress or boost your mood. Each workout is tailored to your energy, mindset, and goals for that day, not anyone else's.

Working out alone also nurtures mental resilience. It's a time to practice focus, to tune into your body, and to quiet any self-doubt. You're not competing with anyone but yourself, allowing you to tap into a space of personal growth, with each workout becoming a small victory in itself.

Building Confidence, One Solo Workout at a Time

One common misconception about solo fitness is that it might leave you feeling isolated or uncertain. But solo workouts offer a unique opportunity to build an unshakable inner confidence. Especially if you're an introvert or just don't like being around the general population. With each session, you're building trust in yourself—trust in your commitment, discipline, and ability to show up consistently for your health and well-being.

At first, working out alone might feel like stepping into unknown territory, especially if you're accustomed to the energy of a gym crowd. However, the quietness of solo fitness is a gift. Here, there are no comparisons, no benchmarks but your own, and no one to judge your progress. Instead, you develop a personal sense of achievement, gaining confidence not from external approval but from witnessing your own growth.

Imagine the pride you'll feel each time you complete a new workout or master a challenging exercise on your own. This confidence transfers beyond the workout itself—it builds resilience and self-assurance that will help you in other areas of life, showing you that you are capable, independent, and determined.

The Advantages of Working Out at Home vs. a Public Gym

The gym is a familiar environment for many, yet it's not always conducive to the focused, personalized experience that solo fitness can offer. When you exercise at home, you're in control of every aspect of your workout environment, from the space to the music, and even the air temperature. This might seem minor, but these small freedoms allow you to fully immerse in the workout without distractions. Sure, you could just show up to the gym when it's not as busy, however that will just make it a pain to schedule and could just lead to a cycle of "I'll do it tomorrow."

Working out at home is just convenient: no commute, no crowds, no need to wait for a machine or clean up after others. I know we've all dealt with the ones that never wipe off the sweat from the bench you've been waiting on. Anyways, you can make your fitness schedule fit seamlessly into your life rather than bending your life around gym hours or other people's routines. This flexibility makes it easier to stay consistent, especially on busy days or when you're less motivated.

Moreover, the privacy of a home workout can lead to a more fulfilling experience, where you feel safe to try new movements and challenge yourself without fear of judgment or distraction. Your space becomes a sanctuary, a place where fitness becomes an intimate act of self-care rather than a chore or obligation.

Moving Forward Together—Independently

This book is your guide to making solo fitness a cornerstone of your well-being, unlocking the mental, emotional, and physical strength that comes from working out alone. You'll discover routines, tips, and motivational strategies that make it easier than ever to pursue your fitness goals from home. Embrace this journey toward self-reliance, confidence, and health. As you step into your solo fitness practice, remember: every movement, every goal reached, is yours alone.

Welcome to a new way of seeing fitness—where your space, peace, and well-being are prioritized. Let's dive in and unlock the incredible potential of solo fitness together.

My Journey with Solo Fitness

Seven years ago, I found myself at a crossroads. I'm sure all, if not most of you, have experienced this. I had been going to the gym for years with close friends, relying on our shared motivation and routines to keep up my fitness goals. But life, as it does, shifted. My friends and I gradually went our separate ways, and I eventually moved to a new area with my new family. The gym lost its familiar faces and energy, and I faced the challenge of maintaining my fitness alone. I only had time for work and spending time with my wife and kids.

I've always been an introvert, and I've always valued my own space and independence, but the shift to solo workouts at home wasn't easy at first. The buzz of a gym replaced by the quiet of my home gym was an adjustment. However, I quickly found that this solitude had its own rewards. Without the distractions of a gym crowd, I was able to connect with my body and my goals in a way I hadn't before. I could focus entirely on myself— my pace, my progress, and my preferences.

At first, I started small, fitting workouts around work, life with two kids, and a busy home. My wife supported me in creating a fitness routine that blended into our family life.Over time, I built a workout routine that gave me not only strength and endurance but also a mental escape and a sense of accomplishment that only grew with each passing year.

Now, fitness has become my time, a break where I can recharge, clear my head, and focus inward. Working out at home allows me the freedom to exercise in a space that feels safe and private. No waiting for equipment, no comparison with others—just me, pushing my limits on my own terms.

In many ways, solo fitness has become my sanctuary, a habit I deeply value. For anyone who's ever felt the need to carve out a personal space in their fitness journey, I hope this guide helps you find your own path.

Chapter 1: Understanding Solo Fitness: Why it works

Breaking Free from Gym Dependency

For many people, the thought of going to the gym is enough to stop them from working out altogether. It's not just a matter of finding the time; it's about navigating an environment that can feel overwhelming, intimidating, or simply inconvenient. If you're someone who feels more hesitant than inspired when stepping into a gym, you're far from alone.

Why Many People Avoid the Gym

The gym might look like the perfect place for fitness, but for many of us, it's a challenging environment. One common reason people avoid the gym is a feeling of "crowd anxiety." Walking into a space packed with people, surrounded by mirrors, and navigating the maze of machines and weights can be intimidating.You might even dread the feeling of being watched and judged, especially if you're just starting. If you are new to fitness, it can also feel more overwhelming, with a sense that everyone else is already an expert. These pressures can add up, turning what should be an energizing experience into one filled with tension or self-consciousness.

And for those who crave privacy and quiet, the gym environment often feels exactly the opposite.

The Frustrations of Waiting and Sharing Equipment

Even if the crowd itself isn't intimidating, waiting for equipment can quickly become a source of frustration. There's nothing like gearing up for a specific workout, only to find that the machine you need is occupied. You wait, try to fill the time with other exercises, and sometimes even lose momentum. I'm sure you've also come across people that lack gym etiquette and just take over the machine or area you have been waiting for. This constant shuffling disrupts the flow of a workout and can leave you feeling discouraged or impatient.

The reality is that gyms, even well-managed ones, often operate at peak capacity, especially during the times most people are free to work out. This leads to constant competition for equipment, creating a level of dependency that's both inconvenient and unnecessary when you consider the freedom of working out at home.

The Challenges of the Gym Environment

Beyond the crowds and equipment, gyms can be loud, bustling spaces filled with background music (sometimes not very good music), clanging weights, and other people's conversations. While some thrive in this atmosphere, others find it distracting. In a gym, it can be hard to tune out the environment, with noise and movement pulling you away from the focus you need for a fulfilling workout. I know you can just put your earbuds in or headphones on, but there's always interruptions that will have you hit pause on your music. From people trying to talk to you or maybe an announcement from employees of the gym, it can be frustrating and distracting.

Privacy is another major factor. It's not easy to feel at ease trying out new exercises or pushing yourself when you're surrounded by others. Many people prefer not to have an audience while they exercise, wanting instead a space where they can be free from judgment or comparison.

Stepping away from the gym means embracing an environment that works for you rather than adjusting yourself to fit the gym's demands. Working out from home offers that flexibility—allowing you to set the pace, tone, and comfort level. This shift not only makes fitness more enjoyable but also more accessible, empowering you to create a consistent, focused workout routine tailored just for you.

The Appeal of Home-Based Fitness

There's a growing appeal to fitness that happens on your terms, in your own space, without the limitations of a public gym. Home-based fitness opens the door to a level of privacy, flexibility, and customization that a gym just can't offer, making it an ideal solution for those who value control over their fitness experience.

Privacy and a Personalized Environment

When you work out at home, you're free from the public eye. There's no one around to watch, no mirrors reflecting every move, and no background noise to pull you away from your focus. This privacy allows you to let go of any self-consciousness and fully invest in your own journey. It's an environment that is yours alone, a place where you can try new exercises, challenge yourself, and build confidence in your abilities without any external pressure.

Beyond the sense of privacy, a home workout space is truly your own. You can design it to meet your needs, whether that means setting up a dedicated corner with weights and resistance bands or simply rolling out a yoga mat in the living room. You control the lighting, the music, and the temperature, crafting an environment that feels comfortable and motivating. This personalized touch allows you to create an atmosphere that not only supports but enhances your workout, making each session something to look forward to.

Time Efficiency: No Commutes, Total Flexibility

One of the greatest benefits of home-based fitness is its time efficiency. When you eliminate the commute to and from the gym, fitness becomes far more accessible and easier to fit into your day. There's no need to factor in travel time or worry about finding parking. Instead, you can focus solely on the workout itself, maximizing every minute and turning fitness into a habit that fits seamlessly into your routine.

With home workouts, you have the freedom to exercise whenever it suits you best—early morning, late at night, or during the kids' nap time. You're not tied to the gym's hours or peak times, which means you can work out at your convenience and energy level. This flexibility can be the difference between sticking to a consistent routine and struggling to make fitness fit around life's demands.

Tailored to Your Comfort and Style

Home-based fitness isn't just convenient; it's adaptable. You can tailor your workouts to your personal preferences, exploring exercises that match your fitness level, interests, and goals. If high-intensity training isn't your style, you can dive into yoga, Pilates, or bodyweight routines. If you're into strength training, resistance bands or dumbbells are easily integrated into a home setup.

This freedom allows you to explore what truly works for you, without the pressure to fit into a "one-size-fits-all" gym environment. You can switch up your routines, experiment with different exercises, or incorporate new forms of movement— all at your own pace. The flexibility to try different workouts in a private, personalized space creates a unique sense of empowerment, making it easier to find what keeps you motivated and energized.

Home-based fitness is more than just a convenient alternative to the gym; it's a lifestyle that honors your individuality. When you work out at home, you're choosing a space that respects your time, comfort, and goals, making each session as enjoyable as it is effective. This is fitness on your terms—empowering, adaptable, and perfectly suited to your life.

Busting Myths About Home Workouts

Home workouts are often misunderstood, clouded by myths that suggest they're less effective or harder to stick with than gym-based routines. But these assumptions miss the full picture. With the right approach and a bit of creativity, home workouts can be powerful, effective, and surprisingly easy to sustain—even in a busy household. Let's break down some common misconceptions that might be holding you back from embracing the full potential of working out at home.

Myth #1: "Home Workouts Don't Deliver Results"

One of the biggest myths about home workouts is that they can't match the intensity or results of a gym routine. This misconception often stems from the idea that home workouts lack the specialized equipment that gyms offer. However, results are driven not by location or fancy machines, but by consistency, effort, and the effectiveness of each movement. The way that I overcame this was by watching videos online. There are many free workout programs on there that show you proper form and recommend starting weights. Just watch what they do and take the time to watch yourself in the mirror until you feel comfortable about your form.

Home-based routines can target every major muscle group and improve strength, flexibility, and endurance—all without the need for bulky equipment. With bodyweight exercises alone, you can achieve incredible gains, from squats and lunges to push-ups and planks. Resistance bands, dumbbells, or even household items can add variety and intensity to your routine, allowing you to progress steadily and achieve powerful results over time. The key is to find a variety of exercises that challenge you and keep your muscles guessing. Mix it up the way you see fit.

Myth #2: "You Need Expensive Equipment to See Progress"

Another misconception is that working out at home requires an elaborate setup with expensive equipment. While it's true that gyms offer a wide range of machines, achieving a balanced and effective workout at home doesn't require much at all. Many fitness goals can be met with just a few key pieces of affordable equipment or even none at all.

Bodyweight exercises like push-ups, squats, and burpees can build strength and endurance without any equipment. For a bit of variety, resistance bands and a pair of dumbbells can be a game-changer, offering a full range of movement and resistance that challenge your muscles in different ways. These compact tools can easily fit into any space, giving you the flexibility to adapt your workouts as you progress. Adjustable weights are for sure a space saver. And if equipment isn't in the cards, you'd be surprised by how effective household items—a chair for tricep dips, a backpack filled with books for added weight—can be in creating a challenging and well-rounded routine.

Myth #3: "It's Harder to Stay Motivated and Disciplined at Home"

There's a common assumption that home workouts are harder to stick to, especially when life's demands—kids, household responsibilities, work—are all around you. While it's true that working out at home requires a certain level of discipline, this can be turned into a strength with the right mindset and approach. Splitting up a workout throughout the day is not a bad thing at all. It's even believed that breaking up your exercise throughout the day can be just as beneficial for your physical and mental health as doing one singular session.

Staying motivated is easier when you view home workouts as a flexible and accessible part of your day. You don't have to carve out large chunks of time; instead, you can fit in a workout when it works best for you, even in shorter sessions. Kids running around? Make it a family activity! Set a playful example and let them join in, or find pockets of time when you can focus, whether early morning, during nap time, or in the evening. Home workouts offer a unique level of adaptability that allows you to prioritize fitness without compromising your daily life.

Ultimately, working out at home builds a form of discipline that's both natural and sustainable. You're learning to rely on yourself for motivation, rather than the environment of a gym or the watchful eyes of others. This kind of self-reliance strengthens not just your body, but your commitment to your own goals—a skill that becomes invaluable as you progress.

Breaking free from these myths opens the door to a world of possibilities in your fitness journey. Home workouts can be as challenging, rewarding, and fulfilling as any gym routine, with the added advantage of being adaptable to your life, family, and personal preferences.

Mindset Shifts for Successful At-Home Workouts

Moving from Gym Dependency to Self-Sufficiency

Going from gym dependency to a self-sufficient fitness routine at home can be transformative. This shift isn't just about changing locations; it's about learning to rely on your own motivation, setting goals that come from within, and developing the discipline to follow through. As you move toward a self-directed fitness journey, you'll find that the rewards go far beyond physical gains. Let's explore how you can build a fitness practice that's truly self-sustaining.

Motivating Yourself Without External Pressures

In a gym, it's common to feel motivated by the people around us, the trainers offering encouragement, or even the buzz of activity. But working out alone teaches you to tap into your own motivations rather than relying on external cues. This can be challenging at first, but the freedom that comes with self-motivation is powerful. Without needing a "boost" from others, you learn to connect more deeply with your reasons for staying active and healthy.

One way to build this motivation is to identify the personal "why" behind your fitness goals. Is it to feel stronger, improve your energy levels, or set an example for your family? Defining what fitness means to you—not to anyone else—fuels the drive to keep going. This self-reflection transforms fitness from an external expectation into an empowering, personal commitment.

Developing Intrinsic Motivation for Lasting Success

Intrinsic motivation is the desire to engage in an activity because of the enjoyment, satisfaction, or sense of accomplishment it brings. When you're intrinsically motivated, fitness becomes more than a task—it becomes a fulfilling part of your life. This internal drive helps you stay consistent, even on the days when motivation is low or life gets busy.

Developing intrinsic motivation means setting goals that genuinely excite you, focusing on the progress and positive feelings that fitness brings. Each workout becomes a small victory, one that you accomplish for your own growth. Over time, this focus on personal rewards helps you build a sustainable relationship with fitness. Instead of exercising to keep up with others, you're doing it because you enjoy the process and are driven by your own progress and goals.

Building Discipline Through Self-Driven Routines

Working out independently requires discipline—a commitment to showing up for yourself consistently. Without the structure of a gym, it can be tempting to skip a workout or let other priorities take over. But building discipline in a home fitness routine is entirely possible, and it begins with creating a regular structure that fits your life.

One effective strategy that I found to work is to schedule workouts as you would any other priority, blocking off specific times that work best for you. By establishing these sessions as part of your routine, they become a natural, expected part of your day. We, as humans, are masters of the routine. Creating simple routines you can rely on is also key. Having a core set of exercises or a go-to workout style means you won't spend time deciding what to do; you can jump right in and keep your momentum strong.

Through self-driven routines, you'll develop a discipline that extends far beyond fitness. This skill—learning to commit to something meaningful for yourself—can impact every area of life, showing you that you have the focus and resilience to achieve your goals independently.

As you make the shift from gym dependency to self-sufficiency, you'll discover that self-motivation, intrinsic rewards, and disciplined routines form the backbone of a lasting fitness journey. This independence not only strengthens your body but also reinforces a confidence in your own ability to set, pursue, and achieve goals—completely on your terms.

Embracing the Process of Self-Improvement

One of the greatest rewards of solo fitness is the journey of self-improvement it creates. When you set out on this path, you're not just aiming for a final destination or a specific result; you're committing to your continuous growth. Embracing this process means setting goals that push you forward, celebrating the small wins along the way, and cultivating patience as you build the fitness level and mindset you want.

Setting Realistic, Incremental Goals for Personal Growth

The key to lasting progress is setting realistic, achievable goals that reflect where you are now and where you'd like to be. Goals don't need to be big or ambitious to be effective—in fact, it's the smaller, manageable targets that often keep you moving forward. Whether it's completing one more rep, running a bit longer, or trying a new movement, each small step brings you closer to a stronger, more resilient self. Become confident in yourself.

Start by focusing on what you can accomplish within the next week or month, even tomorrow. These short-term goals serve as stepping stones, creating a sense of purpose and direction without overwhelming you. By setting these short-term objectives, you build confidence, creating a series of "wins" that keep you engaged and inspired.

Recognizing and Celebrating Small Victories

Every fitness journey is filled with victories, big and small. Too often, we're quick to focus on what's left to achieve rather than acknowledging how far we've come. But taking time to recognize each small win—whether it's holding a plank a little longer, feeling more energized, or just showing up for your workout—can boost your motivation and remind you of the progress you're making.

Celebrating these milestones doesn't require fanfare. It can be as simple as a mental high-five or a moment of gratitude. This practice builds a positive mindset around fitness, shifting the focus from perfection to progress. When you recognize these small steps, you create a fitness journey that's not just about the end result but about the personal growth and joy along the way.

Cultivating Patience and Persistence in Achieving Fitness Objectives

Fitness is a journey of endurance as much as strength or speed. True progress takes time, and patience is essential for building a sustainable fitness habit. Achieving your goals doesn't happen overnight, but with persistence and commitment, each workout adds up to a healthier, more capable you. This long-term approach may be challenging, but it builds resilience, both physically and mentally.

When you encounter setbacks or slower progress than you'd like, remember that consistency is more important than speed. On tough days, a shorter workout or lighter routine still moves you forward. Embrace these moments as part of the journey, knowing that every step, no matter how small, is part of the process. Over time, patience and persistence will become two of your most powerful tools, helping you reach fitness goals that once felt out of reach.

Embracing self-improvement in fitness isn't about racing to a finish line; it's about evolving, growing, and strengthening yourself, one step at a time. By setting incremental goals, celebrating each victory, and nurturing patience, you'll build a journey that honors both your progress and your persistence. Each day, you're creating a fitness practice that's built to last— one that encourages you to keep going, celebrate your wins, and take pride in the person you're becoming. Always remember your "why" for your fitness journey. Let that be the major motivator for you.

Overcoming Common Excuses and Challenges

Starting and maintaining a fitness routine at home can feel intimidating, especially when obstacles—both physical and mental—seem to stand in the way. Yet, with a few strategies and the right mindset, you can overcome these common challenges, ensuring that your journey toward fitness remains strong and steady. Let's look at some of the typical barriers to home fitness and how to work around them.

Identifying and Addressing Potential Barriers

One of the first hurdles many people face with home workouts is a perceived lack of space or equipment. Unlike a gym, which is designed to cater to fitness needs, a home setup often has to be creative. However, effective workouts don't require large areas or extensive gear. A small space—just enough for a yoga mat—is often more than sufficient. Using furniture like chairs for tricep dips or a wall for stability exercises can help you maximize whatever space you have.

As for equipment, fitness goals are fully achievable with minimal tools. Bodyweight exercises, resistance bands, or a set of dumbbells can cover a wide range of movements and muscle groups.I'm not telling you to go out and spend a small fortune on a set of weights or some fancy fitness machine. Just start off simple. For those without equipment, household items like water bottles or backpacks filled with books can substitute for weights.If you have children go ahead and use them as weights too. It will strengthen your bond and possibly get them interested in the importance of fitness. The point is not to let a lack of traditional equipment hold you back. With creativity and flexibility, any space can become a functional workout area.

Overcoming Mental Blocks Around Consistency

Mental barriers, like maintaining motivation or fighting procrastination, can be even more challenging than physical obstacles. When you're working out alone, the responsibility to show up rests solely on you. Without the structure of a gym, it's easy to skip a day or lose momentum. Developing consistency takes a proactive mindset, but there are a few methods to help keep you on track.

Creating a routine with set workout times is one of the most effective ways to establish consistency. Scheduling workouts as you would any other commitment helps make fitness a part of your daily life. Another helpful strategy is to start small; on low-energy days, commit to even a five-minute workout. Once you begin, you may find the motivation to continue longer— but even if you don't, you've reinforced the habit of showing up.

Accountability can also help. Tracking your progress in a journal or app can create a sense of accomplishment and keep you motivated to stay consistent. Consider rewarding yourself for reaching milestones or simply for sticking to your routine. Small incentives and positive reinforcement make the journey feel rewarding and build a habit of consistency over time.

Shifting from an "All or Nothing" Mindset

A common mindset that hinders progress is the idea that workouts must be "all or nothing." This belief can create pressure to always work out at full intensity or to complete a lengthy session. But fitness is a journey, and gradual progress is just as valuable as pushing hard every single time. The last thing you want to do is push too hard and end up hurting yourself.

If you're low on time or energy, it's perfectly fine to scale back. A short stretching session, a quick walk, or a few simple exercises are all steps in the right direction. Embracing a flexible approach helps make fitness sustainable, ensuring you're able to work out consistently without burning out or losing motivation.

Remember that every effort counts. Shifting to a mindset of gradual progress frees you from the stress of perfection, allowing you to celebrate each small step. Fitness isn't about achieving instant results but about creating lasting habits and enjoying the journey.

By recognizing potential obstacles, addressing mental blocks, and embracing gradual progress, you'll find it easier to maintain a consistent and enjoyable home fitness routine. These strategies allow you to focus on progress, not perfection, as you build a sustainable fitness journey that fits seamlessly into your life.

Setting Up Your At-Home Fitness Space

Choosing the Right Space

Creating a dedicated space for your home workouts is an essential step toward building a focused and enjoyable fitness routine. When you choose the right area, you set yourself up for productive sessions that are comfortable, motivating, and safe. Let's explore what to look for in your workout space and how to make it the ideal setting for your fitness journey.

Selecting a Designated Area with Room for Movement

The first step is to find an area with enough room to move freely. While you don't need an entire room, having a designated spot—even a small one—ensures that you're able to stretch, squat, and move without restriction. Ideally, aim for a space where you can lay down a mat and perform exercises without bumping into furniture or walls. For some, this might mean a corner in the living room, a cleared-out section of a bedroom, or even a spot in the garage.

Having a designated workout space, no matter how small, helps create a mental boundary between "workout mode" and the rest of your day. When you enter this area, it's easier to focus and get into the mindset for exercise.

Ensuring Proper Ventilation, Lighting, and Surface

A comfortable workout space requires a few practical essentials. Good ventilation is important, especially for intense sessions. If you can, select a room with a window that can be opened for fresh air or add a fan to keep the area cool and comfortable. A well-ventilated space not only feels better but also helps you sustain energy and avoid overheating.

Lighting is another factor that can impact your motivation and focus. Natural light is ideal, as it energizes and enhances mood, but if that's not possible, opt for bright, consistent lighting that allows you to see your movements clearly. Dim or harsh lighting can be distracting, so aim for a setup that keeps you alert and engaged.

Surface matters, too. Try to work out on a surface that provides enough support and cushioning for your joints. Hard floors are great for stability but can be hard on the body, so consider adding a non-slip exercise mat. This small addition can make a big difference, especially for floor exercises, stretches, and yoga.

Creating a Clutter-Free Environment for Focus and Motivation

Clutter can be a distraction, so aim to keep your workout area organized and free from unnecessary items. When you're not surrounded by unrelated belongings, it's easier to focus on your movements and stay mentally present. If possible, store your equipment neatly in one place, like a small shelf or basket, so it's easy to access but doesn't interfere with your workout flow.

If you're in a multi-purpose space, even a few quick adjustments—like moving distracting items out of view or setting up a small area rug as a visual boundary—can help create a sense of separation. Consider adding small touches that inspire you, like a motivational quote, a mirror, or even a small plant to create a welcoming, personal atmosphere.

Choosing the right space may seem like a small detail, but it can have a huge impact on your home workout experience. With adequate room, proper ventilation and lighting, and a clutter-free environment, you're creating a space that supports both focus and enjoyment. This designated area becomes your personal fitness sanctuary, a place where you can fully invest in your goals and feel motivated to show up every day.

Basic Equipment for Solo Workouts

Starting a home workout routine doesn't mean you need to go out and buy an array of heavy-duty equipment. With a few versatile, space-efficient tools, you can build an effective workout routine that targets every major muscle group and allows for progress over time. Here's how to equip your home workout space to maximize results without overwhelming your space.

Selecting a Designated Area with Adequate Room for Movement

Before diving into equipment, make sure you've designated a space that gives you enough room to move freely. This area should allow for a range of exercises—whether you're lying on a mat, stretching out, or moving side-to-side for a cardio routine. Having a clear, open space helps you move safely and stay focused, ensuring each session is as effective as possible.

Once you have your designated area, you're ready to choose equipment that's both functional and suitable for the space you've carved out.

Investing in Versatile Items: Resistance Bands, Dumbbells, and a Mat

For a comprehensive workout routine at home, a few versatile pieces of equipment can go a long way. Here are some basics I recommend that offer maximum flexibility and adaptability:

- **Resistance Bands**: Lightweight, affordable, and easy to store, resistance bands can enhance nearly any workout. They come in varying levels of resistance, from light to heavy, allowing you to target different muscle groups effectively. Resistance bands are ideal for strength training, stretching, and even mobility exercises, making them one of the most versatile tools for a home workout setup. Make sure to read reviews. We've all seen videos online of them snapping and whipping the person using them. Though it is funny to watch, you do not want to be on the receiving end. Trust me.

- **Dumbbells**: A pair of adjustable dumbbells or a set of lightweight ones can bring variety to your workouts. Start with weights that challenge you without compromising form, then gradually increase as you gain strength. Dumbbells can be used for exercises targeting your arms, legs, core, and more, allowing you to build strength incrementally.

- **Exercise Mat**: A high-quality mat is essential for comfort and support during floor exercises. Whether you're performing core work, stretching, or yoga, a mat provides the right amount of cushioning to protect your joints and enhance stability. Look for a non-slip surface that will stay in place and support you through various types of movements.

These basics allow you to cover a wide range of exercises without taking up much space, making them perfect for solo workouts in any home environment.

Considering Space-Saving Equipment

If you're limited on space but want to expand your workout options, there are some excellent compact tools designed specifically for home setups. Here are a few that offer functionality without taking up much room:

- **Foldable or Adjustable Dumbbells**: Adjustable dumbbells are a fantastic investment for those with limited storage. They allow you to switch between various weight levels within a single compact set, saving both space and money while giving you flexibility for progression.

- **Pull-Up Bar**: A portable pull-up bar that fits in a doorway can provide an effective upper body workout without taking up floor space. Pull-ups, chin-ups, and leg raises are all possible with a sturdy bar, adding variety to your strength routine. Many models are easy to install and remove, making them a space-efficient addition to your home gym. Just make sure to put some towels or even some socks between the foam pads and doorframe. Unless you want those black marks on the frame that are a pain to get off.

- **Kettlebells or Weighted Vest**: If you want to add variety to your resistance training, a kettlebell or weighted vest can offer unique benefits. Kettlebells allow for dynamic, full-body movements, while a weighted vest can intensify bodyweight exercises like squats or push-ups. Both items are compact yet provide a challenging element to your routine.

By selecting equipment that's functional and space-conscious, you're creating a versatile setup that allows you to pursue a full spectrum of fitness goals. From strength and cardio to flexibility and balance, these tools empower you to get the most out of your workouts, all within the comfort of your chosen home space.

With a designated area and a few pieces of versatile equipment, your home becomes a personalized fitness studio, ready to support you in every step of your journey. The beauty of solo workouts lies in their simplicity—no need for crowded spaces or elaborate machines, just a handful of well-chosen tools and the motivation to make each session count.

Creating an Atmosphere that Inspires

Setting up a dedicated, inspiring space for your workouts can have a huge impact on your motivation and enjoyment. When your environment encourages you, workouts feel less like a chore and more like an activity you look forward to. By adding personal, motivating touches, keeping the space clutter-free, and adding an energizing soundtrack, you create a space that makes fitness a positive part of your daily routine. Here's how to craft a workout atmosphere that keeps you inspired.

Using Motivational Cues: Vision Boards, Inspiring Quotes, and Citations

Visual reminders of your goals can be powerful motivators. Consider creating a vision board—a collage of images, quotes, and goals that visually represent your fitness aspirations and the lifestyle you're working toward. Studies show that visualizing your goals can enhance motivation and focus, serving as a constant reminder of the benefits and achievements you're striving for. Quotes can be another effective addition to a workout space. Choose words that resonate with you personally, whether they're reminders to push through challenges, stay consistent, or celebrate progress. You could print quotes and place them on a nearby wall or even write them on a small board where you can see them during workouts. Research suggests that using verbal or visual affirmations can bolster self-belief and increase resilience in achieving goals .

Set Up a Speaker for Energizing or Relaxing Playlists

Music is a powerful motivator, helping you get in the zone and enhancing your workout performance. Set up a speaker or use headphones for playlists that energize or relax you, depending on the type of workout. Upbeat, high-tempo music can boost your endurance and make high-intensity workouts feel more enjoyable, while calming tunes can aid focus during stretching, yoga, or cool-downs . Channel your inner DJ. The energy and flow of your routine; whether it's a pumped-up track to keep you moving or ambient music for a relaxing session, the right soundscape helps you connect with the moment.

Keeping Equipment Organized for a Clean, Welcoming Space

A clutter-free workout space can significantly impact your mindset and motivation. When your equipment is organized, your space feels more open and inviting, allowing you to focus on the workout rather than distractions. Use a small shelf, basket, or wall-mounted hooks to keep items like mats, bands, and dumbbells neatly stored and easy to access. This setup minimizes pre-workout preparation and helps you start each session with a clear mind.

Having a tidy space also supports consistency—when your workout area is well-maintained, it's easier to step into your routine without hesitation. A study on the "impact of your environment" on exercise habits found that organized, aesthetically pleasing spaces can improve adherence to fitness routines by promoting a sense of calm and readiness .

By combining motives, energizing or relaxing playlists, and an organized setup, you're transforming your workout space into a sanctuary of inspiration. This environment isn't just about function; it's about creating a space that reflects your goals, uplifts your spirit, and welcomes you each day to invest in your fitness journey. Whether you're tackling high-intensity moves or unwinding with stretches, an inspiring atmosphere is your foundation for a lasting, positive relationship with fitness.

Chapter 2: The Essentials of Solo Workout Programs

Building a Balanced Routine

Understanding Key Components of Fitness

To create a strong, resilient body, it's important to understand the foundational pillars of fitness: strength, cardio, flexibility, and balance. Each component plays a unique role in supporting a well-rounded and sustainable approach to fitness. By embracing these pillars and balancing your workouts across them, you'll create a routine that not only builds physical capacity but also enhances overall well-being and longevity.

Learning About Strength, Cardio, Flexibility, and Balance as Fitness Pillars

Strength: Strength training focuses on building muscle power and endurance. It's essential for daily function, as stronger muscles support joints, improve posture, and help prevent injury. Whether using body weight, resistance bands, or dumbbells, strength exercises build muscle, improve bone density, and boost metabolism. By working on strength, you're investing in long-term vitality, making everyday tasks easier and preparing your body to withstand physical challenges.

Cardio: Cardiovascular fitness strengthens your heart and lungs, enhancing your body's ability to deliver oxygen to muscles and other tissues. Cardio exercises, from brisk walking and cycling to jumping rope, keep your heart healthy, improve endurance, and help regulate weight. They also have mental benefits, releasing endorphins that reduce stress and elevate mood. Incorporating cardio into your routine can be as simple as taking active breaks throughout the day or dedicating time to more intense aerobic exercises.

Flexibility: Flexibility is often overlooked, but it's a critical component for mobility, injury prevention, and ease of movement. Flexibility exercises, like stretching and yoga, help maintain the range of motion in your joints, reducing stiffness and tension in muscles. Improved flexibility allows for greater freedom in movement, making your strength and cardio exercises more effective and comfortable. It also supports long-term joint health, which is essential for maintaining physical independence as you age.

Balance: Balance training improves stability and body awareness, reducing the risk of falls and enhancing coordination. Balance exercises are particularly useful as we age, but they're valuable at any stage of life, promoting core strength and functional movement. Simple balance exercises, like standing on one leg, planking, or using stability tools, help build core stability and improve control over your body's movements.

Recognizing the Importance of a Holistic Workout Approach

Each fitness pillar contributes something vital to your well-being, but together they form a complete approach to physical health. A holistic fitness routine doesn't just focus on one area; it recognizes that strength, endurance, flexibility, and balance each play essential roles. Embracing all four components helps you avoid imbalances that could lead to discomfort, injury, or limitations in your abilities. By combining these elements, you're developing not only physical strength and stamina but also the capacity to move through life with confidence, resilience, and ease.

Balancing Workouts Across These Components for Well-Rounded Fitness

Finding balance among these fitness components may sound challenging, but it's simpler than you might think. To achieve well-rounded fitness, try dedicating specific days or parts of your workout to different pillars. For example:

- **Strength and Cardio Rotation**: Alternate between strength-focused and cardio-focused days, giving your body time to recover between intensive strength sessions while keeping up cardiovascular endurance.

- **Incorporate Flexibility Daily**: End each workout with stretches to improve flexibility and release tension, or set aside a dedicated day for yoga or longer stretching sessions.

- **Integrate Balance Work**: Add quick balance exercises into your warm-up or cool-down. For instance, single-leg exercises, planks, and core work will naturally improve balance while building strength.

By keeping these pillars in mind, you're setting yourself up for a balanced fitness routine that supports both physical capability and overall health. A comprehensive approach empowers you to feel strong, agile, and resilient, helping you enjoy your fitness journey with a well-rounded, fulfilling outlook on movement.

Structuring Weekly Workout Plans

Building a weekly workout plan is like creating a roadmap for your fitness journey. By structuring your week thoughtfully, you'll set yourself up for steady progress while preventing burnout and ensuring each key fitness component is addressed. A well-rounded plan includes designated focus days, rest and recovery, and flexible timing based on your personal goals and schedule. Here's how to create a weekly workout plan that works for you.

Designating Days for Specific Focuses

Breaking up your week into specific focus areas helps you target different muscle groups, improve various fitness skills, and prevent overuse of any one area. Here's an example of how you might structure your week:

- **Upper Body Days**: Dedicate one or two days each week to upper body strength exercises. Focus on movements like push-ups, rows, and shoulder presses to work the chest, back, arms, and shoulders.

- **Lower Body Days**: Set aside a couple of days for lower body exercises, targeting the legs, glutes, and lower back. Squats, lunges, and glute bridges are excellent choices for building strength in these areas.

- **Cardio Days**: Choose one or two days for cardio-based workouts, where the primary goal is to elevate your heart rate and improve endurance. Cardio could include running, cycling, jump rope, or even high-intensity interval training (HIIT), depending on your goals and preferences.

- **Flexibility and Balance Days**: Dedicate at least one day to flexibility and balance training. This can be a session focused on yoga, Pilates, or deep stretching exercises. Balance exercises like single-leg holds or core planks can be integrated into your strength days, too.

This structure ensures you're hitting every major fitness pillar without overloading any one area, allowing time for recovery while promoting balanced development.

Incorporating Rest Days and Recovery

Rest days are just as important as workout days. They allow your muscles to recover and grow, reduce the risk of injury, and help prevent mental burnout. Aim to include at least one full rest day in your weekly plan, especially if you're doing high-intensity workouts. Some people also benefit from "active recovery" days, where they engage in low-impact activities like walking, stretching, or gentle yoga. These activities keep the blood flowing and support recovery without placing too much stress on the body.

A sample week might look like this:

- **Monday**: Upper Body
  - **Tuesday**: Cardio
  - **Wednesday**: Lower Body
  - **Thursday**: Flexibility and Balance
  - **Friday**: Upper Body (or Cardio if you prefer variety)
  - **Saturday**: Lower Body
  - **Sunday**: Rest or Active Recovery (stretching, walking, etc.)

By allowing time for recovery, you can give each workout your best effort while supporting long-term progress and enjoyment.

Planning Workout Durations Based on Personal Goals and Availability

Your workout durations should be tailored to your goals, current fitness level, and the time you have available. For example:

- **Shorter Sessions** (*20-30 minutes*): If you're short on time or working on building consistency, aim for shorter, intense sessions. HIIT workouts, circuit training, and focused strength routines can be very effective even within 20–30 minutes.

- **Moderate Sessions** (*30-45 minutes*): If your goal is general fitness and health, aim for 30–45 minutes per session. This duration allows you to warm up, complete a solid workout, and include some cool-down stretches without taking up too much of your day.

- **Longer Sessions** (*60+ minutes*): If you have specific goals, like endurance training or advanced strength work, you may benefit from occasional longer sessions. Just be mindful of balancing these longer workouts with adequate recovery time.

Consistency is key, so design a routine that fits smoothly into your life. You can adjust based on energy levels or unexpected events, but having a basic weekly structure will help you stay on track and make steady progress.

By thoughtfully structuring your week, you're setting yourself up for success with a balanced, sustainable plan that promotes strength, endurance, flexibility, and recovery. This approach supports your goals while allowing you to work at a pace that fits your lifestyle, helping you stay motivated and enjoy each step of the journey.

Adapting to Progress and Adjusting Workouts

As you progress on your fitness journey, it's essential to adapt your workouts to reflect your growing strength, endurance, and confidence. When you track your improvements, add new exercises, and keep your routine flexible, you create a workout plan that evolves alongside you, keeping things exciting and challenging. Here's how to ensure your workouts stay effective and engaging as your fitness levels improve.

Track Improvements to Increase Workout Intensity Gradually

Tracking your progress is a motivating way to see just how far you've come. Keeping notes on the weights you lift, the reps you complete, or your cardio endurance can show you where you've improved and where there's room for growth. This record allows you to gradually increase intensity—essential for continued progress. For instance:

- **Strength Training**: If you notice that certain weights feel too light, consider increasing by 5-10% to challenge your muscles more. Alternatively, you can add a few extra reps or sets to extend the workout duration.

- **Cardio**: Track your time, distance, or intensity level. If your 20-minute jog has become easier, try increasing your pace, adding an extra five minutes, or incorporating intervals for an added challenge.

- **Flexibility and Balance**: Track how your range of motion improves or how long you can hold balance poses. Gradually working toward deeper stretches or more complex balancing exercises is a great way to ensure growth.

This gradual increase in intensity, also known as progressive overload, helps you avoid plateaus and keeps your muscles adapting.

Incorporate New Exercises to Prevent Plateaus

Once you become accustomed to a specific set of exercises, your body may stop responding with the same intensity. To keep seeing results, try adding new movements to your routine. Not only does this prevent plateaus, but it also engages different muscles and adds excitement to your workouts. Some ideas include:

- **New Variations**: Change up the variations of exercises you already know. If you're used to standard push-ups, try decline push-ups or diamond push-ups for a new challenge. Replace standard squats with Bulgarian split squats or single-leg squats to work your muscles differently.
- **Different Equipment**: Introduce a new piece of equipment, like kettlebells or resistance bands, to add variety and target different muscle groups. For example, switching from dumbbells to resistance bands offers a unique type of resistance that challenges your muscles in a new way.
- **Cross-Training**: Try different workout styles, like adding a HIIT session if you've been focused on strength or trying a flexibility-based class if you've focused on cardio. Cross-training not only builds a more balanced fitness profile but also keeps workouts enjoyable and varied.

Switching things up regularly can help sustain your progress and reduce the likelihood of mental fatigue.

Maintain Flexibility to Adjust Routines as Fitness Levels Improve

While having a structured plan is important, staying flexible allows you to adapt to changes in your energy levels, interests, or fitness goals. As you become more attuned to your body, you may realize that some workouts need adjusting to keep your routine both challenging and fulfilling. Some ways to stay flexible include:

- **Listen to Your Body**: As you grow stronger, you might find that some workouts feel too easy or even boring. Don't hesitate to modify these sessions to include more complex movements or heavier weights, or switch up the sequence to keep your body guessing.

- **Adjust for Energy Levels**: On days when you're feeling particularly energized, try a more intense or longer workout. Alternatively, if you're low on energy, consider a lighter session focused on flexibility or balance. The ability to pivot based on how you feel can make your routine more sustainable over the long term.

- **Revise Goals as Needed**: Periodically, take a step back to review your goals and make any necessary adjustments. If you originally focused on building strength but now want to increase endurance, shift your plan to incorporate more cardio or interval training. Adapt your routine to fit your evolving objectives, keeping it aligned with what you want to achieve.

By tracking progress, adding new exercises, and staying flexible with your goals, you're creating a dynamic and adaptable fitness journey. This approach keeps workouts fresh, prevents plateaus, and ensures that you continue to challenge yourself as you move forward. Embrace these adjustments, and watch as your progress fuels the confidence and strength you've built over time.

Solo Strength Training at Home

Bodyweight Exercises for Strength

Bodyweight exercises are a powerful and accessible way to build strength without needing complex equipment or a gym. By focusing on foundational moves, progressing to advanced variations, and incorporating compound exercises, you can create a versatile and effective strength routine right at home without weights or equipment. Here's how to get the most out of bodyweight exercises and make steady gains in strength and endurance.

Master Foundational Moves: Squats, Lunges, and Push-Ups

Start by mastering basic movements that lay the groundwork for more advanced exercises. These foundational moves target major muscle groups and help develop stability, balance, and coordination:

- **Squats**: Squats are essential for building lower body strength, targeting your glutes, quads, hamstrings, and core. To perform a squat, stand with feet hip-width apart, push your hips back, and lower down as if sitting in a chair, keeping your chest up and knees tracking over your toes. Strive for that 90 degree angle. Squats also improve mobility and functional strength, helping with everyday activities.

- **Lunges**: Lunges are excellent for isolating each leg, promoting balance and coordination. Start in a standing position, step forward with one foot, and lower your back knee toward the floor, keeping your front knee aligned with your ankle. Lunges primarily work the glutes, quads, and hamstrings while engaging your core for stability.

- **Push-Ups**: Push-ups are a classic upper body and core exercise, working your chest, shoulders, triceps, and core. Start in a plank position, with hands slightly wider than shoulder-width apart. Lower yourself until your chest nearly touches the ground as you breathe in, then push back up as you breathe out. Push-ups can be modified to your strength level, from knee push-ups for beginners to elevated push-ups for more advanced variations.

These exercises form the foundation of a strong body, so focus on proper form and gradually build up your endurance in each.

Progress with Advanced Variations

Once you feel comfortable with the basics, adding advanced variations will increase the challenge and keep your workouts engaging. These variations require greater strength, balance, and control:

- **Single-Leg Squats (Pistol Squats)**: Pistol squats are a challenging single-leg variation that enhances strength, balance, and mobility. Begin by standing on one leg, extending the other leg in front of you, and squatting down while keeping your balance. Single-leg squats work your glutes, quads, and core intensely, making them a great goal for advanced strength. It can be challenging to find the balance for these. Start off by stabilizing yourself with a chair. Just don't rely on it for assistance.

- **Plyometric Push-Ups**: Plyometric push-ups add an explosive element, boosting upper body strength and power. From a standard push-up position, push off the ground forcefully enough that your hands leave the floor, then catch yourself as you lower back down. "Clappers" are just adding a clap of the hands while you're in the air. Just be careful to catch yourself before your face meets the floor. Plyometric movements activate fast-twitch muscle fibers, which are responsible for explosive power.

- **Jump Lunges**: Add a plyometric twist to lunges by incorporating a jump between each step. Start in a lunge position and jump up, switching legs mid-air, and land softly in a lunge with the opposite leg forward. Jump lunges provide a cardio boost while building lower body strength and agility. Be mindful of how much endurance you have in your legs. If you've been working on them and decided to do these while your legs are worn out, just be careful not to try these just to end up on the floor.

Progressing with advanced variations pushes your muscles to adapt, fostering strength and muscle definition while enhancing your coordination and control. As you try different, more dynamic exercises, prioritize your safety and be sure you are ready.

Use Compound Movements to Target Multiple Muscle Groups

Compound exercises are movements that engage multiple muscle groups simultaneously, maximizing efficiency and helping build functional strength. These exercises mimic everyday movements, making them beneficial for overall fitness:

- **Burpees**: Burpees are a full-body exercise that combines a squat, plank, push-up, and jump, targeting the legs, core, chest, and arms. Burpees boost endurance and provide a quick cardio element, making them ideal for high-intensity routines.

- **Mountain Climbers**: This exercise combines core and cardio work, engaging the shoulders, arms, core, and legs. Start in a plank position, then alternate bringing each knee toward your chest as quickly as possible, keeping your core tight and hips low.

- **Bear Crawls**: Bear crawls are a functional movement that involves crawling on all fours, engaging the shoulders, chest, core, and legs. Start in a tabletop position with knees hovering just off the ground, then move forward by stepping with opposite hands and feet. Bear crawls improve coordination, core stability, and upper body strength.

Incorporating compound movements into your routine ensures you're working multiple muscle groups with each exercise, making the most of your time and effort. This approach is highly effective for building balanced strength and endurance while keeping workouts dynamic.

By mastering foundational moves, progressing to advanced variations, and incorporating compound exercises, you're building a bodyweight strength routine that is powerful, adaptable, and rewarding. These exercises are accessible to all fitness levels and require only your body and determination, proving that you don't need a gym to achieve real, sustainable strength.

Adding Resistance with Minimal Equipment

Once you've mastered bodyweight exercises, adding resistance through minimal equipment can significantly boost the intensity of your workouts, helping you build strength, tone muscles, and increase endurance. Resistance bands, dumbbells, and other compact tools offer versatile ways to make your workouts more challenging without requiring a gym. Here's how to safely and effectively incorporate these tools to maximize your solo workout potential.

Use Resistance Bands or Dumbbells for Added Intensity

Resistance bands and dumbbells are compact, affordable options that add resistance and variety to your exercises, targeting different muscle groups more effectively.

- **Resistance Bands**: These bands come in various levels of resistance, from light to heavy, allowing you to adjust intensity as you progress. Resistance bands are excellent for exercises like squats, bicep curls, and lateral band walks. They're also gentle on joints and versatile enough to be used in various movement patterns, making them a great option for a full-body workout.

- **Dumbbells**: Dumbbells provide stable weight, enabling you to add resistance incrementally and control movement more precisely. With just a couple of sets (or even adjustable dumbbells), you can increase the challenge of exercises like lunges, rows, or overhead presses. Dumbbells engage stabilizing muscles, encouraging a more comprehensive workout that improves both strength and coordination.

Both resistance bands and dumbbells allow you to progressively overload your muscles—essential for continued growth—while keeping your setup simple and efficient.

Learn Safe Techniques for Common Exercises

When using weights, form is crucial to prevent injury and ensure you're targeting the right muscles. Here's a quick guide to a few fundamental exercises:

- **Bicep Curls**: Stand with feet hip-width apart, holding a dumbbell in each hand at your sides. Keep elbows close to your torso and curl the weights up toward your shoulders, then lower back down with control. Avoid swinging or using momentum to lift the weights; the movement should be slow and steady.

- **Shoulder Press**: Hold a dumbbell in each hand at shoulder height, with palms facing forward and elbows bent. Press the weights overhead until your arms are fully extended, then slowly lower them back down. Keep your core engaged to protect your back and avoid arching as you press upward.

- **Squats with Resistance Bands**: Place the band around your thighs just above the knees, and stand with feet hip-width apart. Perform a standard squat, pressing your knees outward to maintain tension in the band. This extra resistance works your glutes and outer thighs more intensely.

By focusing on proper technique, you'll not only prevent injury but also ensure that each exercise is as effective as possible, helping you to see results sooner.

Explore Alternative Equipment like Kettlebells or Weighted Vests

If you're ready to vary your resistance training further, kettlebells and weighted vests offer unique ways to intensify your workouts without bulky or complex equipment.

- **Kettlebells**: Kettlebells are compact weights with a handle that allow for dynamic, multi-directional exercises, such as swings, cleans, and Turkish get-ups. The offset weight of a kettlebell challenges your stabilizing muscles, building core strength and improving coordination. Kettlebell exercises often combine cardio and strength, making them ideal for high-intensity interval workouts.

- **Weighted Vests**: Weighted vests add uniform weight to your body, making bodyweight exercises like push-ups, lunges, or squats more challenging without the need for holding weights. This type of equipment is perfect if you want to add resistance but keep your hands free, and the added weight enhances endurance and strength over time.

Both kettlebells and weighted vests are versatile options for solo workouts and can easily fit into a home workout routine, allowing for a wide range of movement while building strength.

Adding resistance to your routine with minimal equipment brings a powerful edge to home workouts. Whether you're incorporating resistance bands, dumbbells, kettlebells, or a weighted vest, each piece of equipment enables you to increase intensity and continue challenging yourself in new ways. By learning safe techniques and experimenting with different equipment, you can tailor your workouts to suit your goals, pushing your strength to new levels without needing a gym setup. Just don't break the bank. Invest in these as you continue your fitness journey.

Progressive Overload in Home Workouts

Progressive overload is a powerful principle in strength training that involves gradually increasing the demand on your muscles to keep them growing and adapting. In a home workout setting, where heavy equipment may be limited, it's still entirely possible to apply this principle by creatively adjusting factors like reps, sets, tempo, and resistance. Here's how to keep your home workouts challenging, efficient, and continuously effective as you build strength over time.

Increase Reps, Sets, or Resistance as Strength Improves

One of the simplest ways to incorporate progressive overload is by increasing the volume of your workout as you get stronger. By gradually adding more reps or sets to your exercises, or increasing the resistance you're working against, you're ensuring your muscles are consistently challenged:

- **Reps and Sets**: If you're performing push-ups and find you can do 10 comfortably, try adding a few more reps each session or increasing the number of sets. Small, incremental increases over time help build endurance and strength while allowing your body to adjust gradually.

- **Resistance**: If you're using weights, start with a manageable load, and aim to increase it by a small percentage as you progress. For those using resistance bands, switch to a band with higher resistance once the exercises feel too easy. Increasing resistance, even slightly, keeps your muscles working harder and promotes growth.

Increasing reps, sets, or resistance as your strength improves allows for consistent progress without a drastic change in your routine.

Experiment with Tempo Changes

Altering the tempo of your movements, particularly by slowing down the eccentric (or lengthening) phase, can significantly increase the challenge of any exercise. This technique doesn't require more weight or reps—just a more mindful, controlled approach to movement:

- **Slow Eccentric Movements**: For exercises like squats or push-ups, slow down as you lower yourself, taking three to four seconds to reach the bottom position. This longer eccentric phase increases the time your muscles are under tension, creating greater fatigue and promoting strength and muscle growth.

- **Pausing at the Bottom**: Another tempo change is to pause at the bottom of a movement (e.g., holding a squat at the lowest point for a few seconds before coming back up). These pauses add an extra challenge for your muscles and help develop control and stability.

Tempo changes can make bodyweight exercises more intense without the need for additional equipment. Plus, they improve control, form, and muscular endurance.

Track Weights or Resistance Levels to Ensure Consistent Progress

Tracking your workouts allows you to measure your progress and set realistic, achievable goals. Whether you're using weights, resistance bands, or simply tracking your reps, having a record of your progress gives you a clear picture of how far you've come and where you want to go:

- **Log Weights or Resistance Levels**: If you're using equipment like dumbbells or kettlebells, note the weight you're lifting for each exercise. Write down the reps and sets as well, so you can see when you're ready to increase the weight or add another set.

- **Track Bodyweight Progressions**: Even without weights, you can track progress by noting how many reps of each exercise you're completing or how long you're holding specific movements. For example, if you start with 10 push-ups and are later able to complete 20, you have a concrete sign of improvement.

- **Set Short-Term Goals**: Based on your records, set incremental goals to push yourself forward. These might be adding one more rep each week or increasing the resistance band strength every month. Setting small goals keeps you motivated and helps you avoid plateaus.

Keeping track of your progress doesn't just show you where you're improving; it also gives you an opportunity to celebrate your achievements, no matter how small, and keep challenging yourself further.

Applying progressive overload in home workouts is a practical and effective way to build strength and endurance over time. By gradually increasing reps, sets, or resistance, experimenting with tempo changes, and tracking your progress, you can continue to challenge your muscles and achieve consistent improvement—all without needing a full gym setup. Progressive overload keeps your workouts dynamic and rewarding, proving that even in a home setting, you can continually push your limits and achieve lasting strength.

Effective Cardio Without a Treadmill

High-Intensity Interval Training (HIIT)

High-Intensity Interval Training (HIIT) is a powerful workout strategy that combines short bursts of intense exercise with brief rest periods, maximizing cardiovascular and metabolic benefits in minimal time. HIIT is ideal for home workouts because it requires little to no equipment, keeps your heart rate elevated, and can be adapted to any fitness level. Here's how to design a simple, high-energy HIIT routine that delivers big results.

Design Simple, High-Energy Circuits

HIIT circuits are meant to be straightforward and engaging, focusing on movements that target multiple muscle groups while keeping your energy high. Choose exercises that can be performed quickly and with intensity, using your body weight or minimal equipment:

- **Sample HIIT Circuit**: A basic routine could include 30 seconds each of burpees, jump squats, mountain climbers, and high knees, followed by a 30-second rest. Repeat this circuit three to five times, depending on your fitness level.

- **Compound Movements**: Opt for exercises that work several muscle groups simultaneously, like burpees (which engage the legs, core, and upper body) and jump squats (which target the glutes, quads, and calves). Compound exercises boost calorie burn and create a full-body workout in less time.

- **Timed Intervals**: You can adjust interval times to fit your fitness level, such as 20 seconds of work followed by 10 seconds of rest for beginners, or 45 seconds on, 15 seconds off for more advanced exercisers.

Keeping your HIIT circuits simple makes them easy to follow and maintain at a high intensity, ensuring that each movement is effective without complicated choreography or equipment.

Keep Sessions Short but Intense for Maximum Cardiovascular Benefits

One of the main advantages of HIIT is its efficiency. Because HIIT is performed at near-maximal effort, sessions can be much shorter than traditional workouts while still delivering impressive benefits for cardiovascular health, calorie burn, and endurance:

- **Effective Time Frame**: Most HIIT workouts last between 10 and 20 minutes, making it easy to fit into any schedule. These brief sessions pack a punch, providing the equivalent of longer, moderate-intensity workouts in less time.

- **Afterburn Effect**: HIIT stimulates excess post-exercise oxygen consumption (EPOC), also known as the "afterburn" effect. This means that even after you finish the workout, your body continues burning calories at an elevated rate as it returns to its normal state.

- **Improved Cardiovascular Health**: The high intensity of HIIT improves heart health by increasing your VO_2 max (the maximum amount of oxygen your body can use during intense exercise), which is a key indicator of cardiovascular fitness. Regular HIIT workouts can reduce blood pressure, lower cholesterol, and improve circulation.

By keeping your HIIT sessions short and intense, you maximize cardiovascular benefits, allowing you to make the most of your time and energy in a quick, high-reward workout.

Allow Adequate Rest for Effective Recovery

HIIT can be demanding on your muscles and cardiovascular system, so it's essential to include adequate rest both within the workout and between sessions to promote recovery:

- **Rest Intervals**: In each circuit, balance your work periods with brief rest intervals, such as 30 seconds of rest between rounds. This allows your heart rate to decrease slightly and gives your muscles a quick recovery window, enabling you to maintain high intensity throughout the workout.

- **Recovery Days**: Avoid doing HIIT every day; your muscles need time to repair, and your nervous system benefits from lower-intensity days. Aim for two to three HIIT sessions per week and incorporate lighter, lower-impact workouts or rest days in between to support full recovery.

- **Listen to Your Body**: As HIIT workouts are intense, it's crucial to recognize when your body needs more rest. If you feel unusually fatigued or sore, take an extra day to recover before your next high-intensity session.

Proper recovery not only prevents burnout and injury but also ensures that each HIIT workout is as effective as possible, keeping your energy high and your performance consistent.

HIIT offers a powerful and efficient workout option that combines high-intensity circuits, short duration, and effective rest periods to build cardiovascular strength and burn calories in a fraction of the time. By designing simple circuits, maintaining intensity, and allowing for adequate recovery, you can harness the benefits of HIIT from the comfort of home, giving you a robust, energizing workout that fits seamlessly into your solo fitness routine.

Low-Impact Cardio Options

Low-impact cardio exercises offer an effective way to improve cardiovascular fitness while being gentle on the joints, making them ideal for anyone with joint concerns or those looking for a less jarring alternative to high-impact movements. With the right approach, low-impact cardio can still provide a challenging workout, enhancing endurance, strength, and overall cardiovascular health without the need for intense jumping or heavy impact on the body. Here's how to build a solid low-impact cardio routine that keeps your heart rate up and your body engaged.

Practice Lower-Impact Moves

Low-impact cardio doesn't have to mean low energy. By choosing movements that are grounded but still dynamic, you can maintain an effective workout that keeps your heart pumping and muscles working:

- **Marches**: Marching in place with high knees is a simple yet effective way to increase heart rate. Lift each knee as high as possible and swing your arms to add intensity. This movement is especially beneficial for warming up or for anyone seeking a gentle cardio option.

- **Step-Ups**: Using a sturdy step or platform, alternate stepping up and down, engaging your glutes, quads, and calves. Step-ups are great for building lower body strength while keeping the movement grounded, and they can be performed at a faster pace to increase cardio intensity.

- **Shadow Boxing**: Shadow boxing is a high-energy, low-impact cardio option that involves throwing controlled punches while moving your body in place. It works the upper body, improves coordination, and increases heart rate without any jumping. Keep your stance active, moving from side to side or adding small squats to incorporate the lower body as well.

By focusing on grounded yet dynamic exercises like marches, step-ups, and shadow boxing, you'll create a high-energy workout without stressing your joints.

Modify Exercises to Accommodate Joint or Mobility Needs

Low-impact cardio is highly adaptable, allowing you to tailor movements to accommodate joint sensitivity or mobility needs without compromising intensity:

- **Range of Motion Adjustments**: Adjust movements to a range that feels comfortable for you. For example, if full squats are challenging, try half squats, which can reduce strain on the knees. Similarly, a gentle lunge instead of a deep lunge can ease joint stress.

- **Supportive Equipment**: Using a wall, chair, or railing for support can improve stability during exercises like step-ups or lateral leg raises, particularly if you're easing into fitness or working on balance.

- **Lower Body-Weight Pressure**: Moves like stationary

marches or standing knee lifts offer effective cardio without putting undue pressure on your knees or ankles, making them ideal options for a safe, low-impact workout.

The ability to modify exercises gives you control over the intensity and makes low-impact cardio suitable for all fitness levels, especially for those mindful of joint health.

Maintain Intensity Through Consistent, Controlled Movements

One of the keys to effective low-impact cardio is maintaining steady, controlled movements. Consistent pacing ensures that you're reaping the cardiovascular benefits without relying on high impact:

- **Controlled Reps**: Perform each rep with purpose, maintaining good posture and engaging your muscles. In shadow boxing, for example, concentrate on strong, deliberate punches rather than speeding through the motions. Quality reps at a moderate pace are more effective than rushing through without control.

- **Keep the Core Engaged**: By keeping your core muscles engaged, you'll maintain stability and enhance overall strength. This also protects your lower back during moves like step-ups or side lunges, where balance and core support are essential.

- **Pacing and Rhythm**: Try to maintain a rhythm that allows you to stay active for a set duration without needing to stop frequently. For instance, alternate between moves like step-ups and marches for one-minute intervals, creating a steady, active flow that boosts cardiovascular endurance over time.

Low-impact cardio can be as intense and beneficial as high-impact routines when performed with consistency and control, allowing you to elevate your heart rate and build fitness without stressing the joints.

Low-impact cardio options are an excellent way to improve cardiovascular health, especially for those who want to prioritize joint safety or prefer a gentler workout style. By incorporating grounded movements, adjusting exercises for comfort, and maintaining a steady, controlled intensity, you can enjoy a powerful and effective cardio session that fits seamlessly into your solo fitness routine, ensuring you're able to keep moving, building endurance, and staying motivated at your own pace.

Incorporating Cardio with Limited Space

When working out in a small space, you can still achieve a high-quality cardio session with compact, effective exercises and a little creativity. By focusing on movements that don't require much room, using what's available (like stairs), and designing routines specifically for limited areas, you'll make the most of your workout environment and keep your heart rate up without the need for a gym or large workout area.

Use Compact Movements

Compact cardio exercises are ideal for small spaces, allowing you to stay active without moving around much. These movements keep your body energized and engaged while minimizing the need for lateral or expansive movements:

- **Jumping Jacks**: A staple of any cardio routine, jumping jacks can be done in place, engaging the entire body and providing a quick way to increase heart rate. For a lower-impact option, step out one foot at a time instead of jumping.

- **Mountain Climbers**: This high-intensity exercise doesn't require much room but provides a full-body workout and increases cardiovascular endurance. Perform mountain climbers in a plank position and bring one knee toward your chest at a time, alternating quickly to keep up the intensity.

- **High Knees**: Stand in place and bring each knee up toward your chest in a rapid, running-in-place motion. High knees are great for boosting cardio while targeting the core, legs, and hip flexors.

Compact movements like jumping jacks, mountain climbers, and high knees are perfect for small spaces and provide a powerful cardio workout without requiring much room to move around.

Take Advantage of Stairs for Added Intensity

If you have access to stairs, they can be an excellent tool for increasing cardio intensity and incorporating a range of exercises that target the lower body:

- **Stair Runs or Walks**: Simply running or walking up and down the stairs provides an intense cardio workout, building strength in your legs and improving cardiovascular health. Adjust the speed and number of steps you take to vary the intensity.

- **Step-Ups and Box Jumps**: Use the bottom step for step-ups or box jumps if it's sturdy. This adds a strength component to your workout, targeting the glutes, quads, and calves while keeping your heart rate up.

- **Stair Lunges**: Perform lunges on the stairs, placing one foot on the first or second step and lowering yourself in a controlled motion. This variation is effective for strengthening the lower body, particularly the quads and hamstrings, while adding a cardiovascular element.

Using stairs adds a level of challenge and intensity to your workout, making even a limited area feel like a functional fitness space with plenty of options for cardio and strength.

Design Space-Saving Routines

You don't need a large area to complete an effective cardio routine. By focusing on space-efficient exercises and circuit-style routines, you can create a dynamic workout that fits your surroundings:

- **Stationary Circuit**: Design a circuit that includes exercises like burpees, squats, high knees, and mountain climbers. Perform each movement for 30 seconds with 10–15 seconds of rest between them, creating a high-intensity, low-space workout.

- **Tabata-Style Workouts**: Tabata intervals (20 seconds of intense exercise followed by 10 seconds of rest) work well in a small space and can include compact moves like jump squats, speed punches, and side lunges. This setup keeps you moving and elevates your heart rate in a short amount of time.

- **Resistance Bands and Bodyweight Movements**: Incorporate resistance bands to add variety without needing much room. Moves like banded marches, lateral leg raises, and shadow boxing with bands can make a small-space workout more challenging.

Designing space-saving routines allows you to get creative with your cardio and fit a complete workout into any limited area, maximizing intensity while keeping movement compact and efficient.

By incorporating compact movements, utilizing stairs, and designing routines that work within your available space, you can achieve a versatile and effective cardio workout even in the smallest of areas. These strategies allow you to maintain consistency and intensity without feeling limited by your environment, proving that a great cardio workout is possible anywhere—no large gym floor required.

Chapter 3: Staying Motivated in Solo Fitness

Goal Setting and Tracking Progress

Setting SMART Fitness Goals

Setting clear, well-defined goals is one of the most powerful tools in achieving long-term fitness success. SMART goals—Specific, Measurable, Achievable, Relevant, and Time-bound—provide a structured framework that helps turn your fitness aspirations into actionable steps. This method not only helps keep you focused but also boosts motivation and provides a sense of accomplishment as you track your progress.

Define Specific, Measurable, Achievable, Relevant, and Time-bound Goals

The SMART goal-setting framework is designed to bring clarity and direction to your fitness journey. By applying each element, you'll ensure your goals are realistic and aligned with your personal growth:

- **Specific**: Your goal should be clear and precise. Instead of setting a vague goal like "get fit," aim for something specific, such as "increase my bench press by 20 pounds" or "run 3 miles without stopping." The more detailed the goal, the easier it is to focus on.

- **Measurable**: Define a clear way to track your progress. This might involve tracking distance, time, repetitions, or even changes in how your body feels during exercise. For example, "lose 10 pounds in 3 months" or "do 10 push-ups in a row" are measurable targets.

- **Achievable**: While it's important to set challenging goals, they must also be realistic. Assess your current fitness level and ensure your goals are within reach. Starting with small, attainable objectives will build your confidence as you progress.

- **Relevan**t: Your goals should align with your values and fitness aspirations. Think about why you're working toward a particular goal. If you're aiming for better cardiovascular health, then running or cycling might be relevant, while strength training might align more with your goals if you're seeking muscle gain.

- **Time-bound**: Set a deadline for achieving your goal. This creates urgency and provides structure, whether it's a short-term goal (such as "complete 30-minute workouts 3 times a week for the next month") or a long-term target (like "reach my target weight by the end of the year").

By creating SMART goals, you provide yourself with a clear blueprint for success, making it easier to stay focused and motivated along your fitness journey.

Break Down Large Goals into Smaller, Manageable Steps

While big goals are motivating, they can also feel overwhelming if they aren't broken down into smaller, actionable steps. By dividing a larger goal into mini-goals, you make the process more manageable and enjoyable:

- **Step-by-Step Progression**: If your goal is to run a 5K, break it into phases, such as starting with walking 10 minutes daily, then progressing to jogging 1 mile, and eventually running 5 kilometers. These incremental steps give you a sense of accomplishment at each stage.

- **Weekly or Monthly Milestones**: Set smaller benchmarks that you can check off along the way. If your goal is to lose weight, aim for losing 1–2 pounds per week, or if you want to improve strength, focus on adding a few extra reps or weight to your routine each week.

- **Adjust as Needed**: Sometimes, progress doesn't always follow the path we envision. Don't be afraid to adjust your smaller goals if you find you need more time or a different approach. Flexibility allows you to stay on track without feeling discouraged.

Breaking larger goals down into smaller, bite-sized pieces helps you stay motivated, boosts your confidence with each achievement, and prevents you from feeling overwhelmed by the bigger picture.

Reflect on Goals Weekly or Monthly for Added Motivation

Reviewing your goals regularly is key to staying motivated and making adjustments when necessary. Consistent reflection helps keep your goals front and center and provides an opportunity to track your progress:

- **Weekly Check-Ins**: Every week, assess your progress. Are you on track to hit your targets? Are there any challenges that need to be addressed? Weekly reflection can help you tweak your routine, make small changes, and stay accountable to your fitness journey.

- **Monthly Progress Reviews**: At the end of each month,

take a broader view. Look at your overall progress, celebrate milestones, and evaluate what's working well or what might need improvement. If you're behind on a goal, this is the perfect time to reassess and set new strategies to get back on track.

- **Celebrate Achievements**: Take time to recognize and celebrate your progress, even the small wins. Whether it's completing a workout challenge, reaching a new personal best, or simply sticking to your routine for the month, acknowledging your success helps fuel motivation to keep going.

Regular reflection is not just about tracking progress—it's also about giving yourself credit for the hard work and determination you've put into your fitness goals. This encourages a positive mindset and fuels further motivation.

Setting SMART fitness goals is a powerful way to ensure you stay on track, measure your progress, and continue to challenge yourself in a structured way. Breaking your goals down into manageable steps and reflecting on your progress regularly helps maintain motivation and creates a clear path to success. With a SMART goal approach, you'll have a strong foundation for your fitness journey, turning aspirations into tangible achievements and ensuring consistent progress along the way.

Tracking and Celebrating Milestones

In any fitness journey, tracking your progress and celebrating milestones play essential roles in keeping motivation high and fostering a sense of accomplishment. These practices help you stay connected to your goals, visualize your improvements, and reinforce the hard work you're putting in. By recording progress, taking regular measurements, and rewarding yourself for reaching milestones, you create a powerful cycle of progress and positive reinforcement that makes it easier to stay committed over the long haul.

Record Progress in a Fitness Journal or App

A fitness journal or app serves as a dedicated space for recording your journey, from daily workouts to weekly reflections and monthly milestones. Documenting progress allows you to see where you started and how far you've come, helping you stay motivated and mindful of every achievement, big or small.

- **Fitness Journal**: Use a notebook or printed template to log each workout, tracking details like exercises, sets, reps, and any personal notes on how you felt or adjustments made. Many people also include sections for nutrition, daily mood, or energy levels, which helps provide insight into how different factors impact their performance.

- **Fitness Apps**: Digital tools like MyFitnessPal, JEFIT, or

Strava allow for easy logging and tracking of activities, calories, and other metrics. Apps often include built-in reminders and progress charts to help visualize your achievements over time, plus the convenience of tracking on-the-go (MyFitnessPal, 2023; Strava, 2023).

- **Sample Entry**: For example, a simple journal entry might read: "Monday – Squats: 3 sets of 12, Push-ups: 3 sets of 10, Plank: 1 min hold. Felt strong, increased reps by 2." This lets you look back at past entries to monitor improvements, identify patterns, and set new goals.

Recording progress keeps you accountable and focused, providing both a clear record of your journey and a personal space to reflect on your experiences and celebrate each step forward.

Take Monthly Photos or Measurements to Visualize Changes

Seeing physical progress can be one of the most rewarding aspects of a fitness journey. Taking monthly photos or measurements offers a visual representation of your hard work, showing changes in muscle tone, posture, and even confidence. It's often easier to notice these changes over time, helping to boost motivation and solidify your commitment.

- **Monthly Photos**: Stand in the same spot, wearing similar clothing each month to keep the focus on physical changes. Capture front, side, and back views to document visible progress. This consistent practice helps you notice gradual changes that may not be as noticeable day-to-day.

- **Measurements**: Use a measuring tape to track areas like arms, chest, waist, hips, and thighs. These measurements can reveal progress even when the scale doesn't, providing a more comprehensive view of how your body is transforming.

- **Tracking Non-Physical Changes**: Beyond the visual, pay attention to how you feel. Improved posture, increased energy, or better stamina during workouts are also meaningful progress markers, even if they're not as obvious in photos or measurements.

Monthly photos and measurements create a tangible record of progress and help maintain motivation, allowing you to appreciate the cumulative effects of your dedication.

Reward Yourself for Meeting Specific Milestones

Reaching a fitness milestone deserves celebration. Setting rewards for specific achievements—whether it's a new personal best, a weight goal, or consistent attendance—helps reinforce positive behavior and makes the journey more enjoyable. Rewards can be anything that brings joy and encourages you to keep moving forward.

- **Non-Food Rewards**: Treat yourself to a new piece of workout gear, a massage, a book, or a day off to relax and recharge. These types of rewards support your fitness goals and enhance your experience.

- **Experience-Based Rewards**: Plan something special, like a day hike, a fun fitness class, or a small trip, as a way to celebrate milestones. Experiences offer a memorable reward that reinforces your dedication and lets you enjoy the results of your hard work.

- **Smaller Rewards for Consistency**: Reward yourself even for hitting smaller consistency goals, like completing a month of workouts or sticking to a new routine. This type of positive reinforcement builds motivation, as you get to experience frequent, small successes along the way.

By celebrating your milestones, you create a positive loop where achievements lead to rewards, boosting your enjoyment and satisfaction with each step of the journey.

Tracking and celebrating your fitness progress are crucial steps in maintaining long-term commitment and motivation. Using a journal or app, taking regular photos and measurements, and setting rewards for your achievements keep you connected to your goals and provide encouragement along the way. Together, these practices create a powerful cycle of motivation, helping you stay focused on your fitness journey and appreciate each milestone you reach.

Adjusting Goals as Fitness Levels Improve

As you progress in your fitness journey, your goals should evolve along with your growing strength, stamina, and capabilities. Recognizing your achievements and setting new challenges keeps your workouts engaging, fosters continuous growth, and helps prevent plateaus. Adjusting goals allows you to add fresh elements to your routine, cater to your evolving interests, and keep your body and mind engaged over the long term.

Recognize Progress and Shift to More Challenging Goals

Acknowledging how far you've come in your fitness journey is both motivating and empowering. Recognize the improvements you've made—whether it's lifting heavier, running longer, or simply feeling more confident. Use these achievements as a foundation to set new, more challenging goals that push your limits and inspire continued growth.

- **Reflect on Your Progress**: Review your initial goals and assess what you've achieved. For example, if your original aim was to do 10 push-ups, but you're now easily doing 15, it's time to raise the bar. Reflecting on your accomplishments keeps you motivated and shows you what's possible.

- **Set New Challenges**: Consider increasing the difficulty by aiming for more reps, heavier weights, or faster times. Or, if you've been working on endurance, try adding strength or power-focused goals to balance your capabilities and broaden your fitness.

- **Keep it Balanced**: Balance challenging goals with achievable steps so they're both motivating and realistic. This way, you'll keep pushing yourself without feeling overwhelmed.

Shifting your goals as you make progress keeps your fitness journey fresh and allows you to continue building on the solid foundation you've created.

Add New Fitness Elements

Expanding your fitness routine to include new components not only keeps things interesting but also contributes to a well-rounded fitness profile. Incorporating endurance, flexibility, balance, or mobility exercises provides variety, prevents overuse injuries, and enhances your overall strength and resilience.

- **Endurance Training**: If you've mainly focused on strength, consider adding cardio sessions to build endurance. This might mean integrating HIIT sessions, cycling, or longer runs. Endurance adds a valuable dimension to your routine, enhancing stamina and cardiovascular health.

- **Flexibility and Mobility**: Introducing flexibility work, like yoga or targeted stretching, helps improve range of motion, reduce muscle tightness, and prevent injuries. Flexibility is often overlooked but is a key component of long-term fitness and mobility.

- **Balance and Stability**: Core stability and balance exercises, such as single-leg work or stability ball exercises, help enhance coordination and core strength. Improved balance reduces the risk of falls and improves performance in other types of exercises.

Adding these new elements not only enhances your physical abilities but also keeps your workouts dynamic, preventing monotony and encouraging comprehensive fitness growth.

Stay Adaptable to Evolving Needs and Interests

As your life and interests evolve, so should your fitness routine. Being flexible and open to change lets you adapt to new challenges, pursue new fitness passions, and find joy in different types of movement. Whether it's due to a lifestyle change, a new fitness interest, or a need for something fresh, adaptability is key to sustaining long-term engagement.

- **Adjust for Lifestyle Changes**: Life events—like changes in schedule, family commitments, or even energy levels— may require shifts in your workout routine. Embrace these adjustments as part of your fitness journey. For example, if time becomes limited, explore shorter, high-intensity workouts to maintain fitness.

- **Explore New Interests**: Maybe you've developed a new interest in hiking, swimming, or martial arts. Introducing new activities allows you to stay excited about working out and builds diverse skills. This variety ensures you're continuously learning, growing, and challenging yourself in fresh ways.

- **Reassess Goals Regularly**: Schedule periodic reviews of your fitness goals and make changes as needed. Evolving your goals according to what you enjoy and what challenges you will help sustain motivation and ensure your workouts remain both effective and fulfilling.

Adaptability allows you to honor where you are in your fitness journey and make adjustments that support your growth, balance, and enjoyment over time.

By recognizing your progress, adding new fitness elements, and staying adaptable, you keep your fitness journey engaging and forward-focused. Adjusting your goals as your abilities improve ensures that your routine evolves with you, keeping things fresh, challenging, and meaningful. As you continue to progress, remember to celebrate how far you've come while staying excited for all the new goals yet to be achieved.

Staying Consistent Without a Gym Routine

Building a Routine That Fits Your Life

Creating a fitness routine that seamlessly fits into your daily life is key to staying consistent and achieving long-term success. When your workout schedule aligns with your natural rhythms and daily activities, it feels less like a chore and more like a fulfilling part of your day. By identifying optimal times, pairing workouts with everyday routines, and setting reminders, you can develop a structure that encourages consistency and reduces the likelihood of skipping sessions.

Identify Optimal Workout Times and Stick to Them

Finding the best time for your workouts can make a significant difference in maintaining a routine. Whether you're an early riser or feel more energized later in the day, aligning your workouts with your natural preferences helps you stick with them in the long term.

- **Experiment with Different Times**: Try morning, afternoon, and evening workouts to see what feels best for your energy levels and schedule. If mornings suit you, a quick session before your day begins can set a positive tone. If you have more energy after work, an evening workout might be the perfect way to decompress.

- **Consistency is Key**: Once you've identified your optimal workout time, commit to it as much as possible. Having a set schedule helps establish a habit, making it easier to stick with your routine over time. Treat this time as a non-negotiable appointment with yourself.

- **Adapt When Needed**: Life can throw surprises, so it's okay to be flexible when things come up. If you miss a morning session, try to fit it in later in the day. The important part is making a habit of showing up for yourself regularly.

Identifying and sticking to an optimal time makes working out feel like a natural part of your day, increasing the likelihood that you'll stay committed.

Pair Workouts with Daily Activities for Seamless Integration

Integrating workouts with existing daily habits can help you create a routine that feels effortless. Pairing exercise with daily activities provides structure and helps make fitness an integral part of your lifestyle rather than an isolated task.

- **Link to a Regular Activity**: Attach your workout to a daily habit, like exercising after your morning coffee or before dinner. This creates a natural cue for exercise, reinforcing the habit. For example, if you start with a few minutes of stretching before breakfast, it becomes part of your morning routine.

- **Incorporate Active Breaks**: Use short exercise breaks during other daily activities. If you work from home, for example, try doing a quick set of squats or push-ups between meetings or using part of your lunch break for a brisk walk.

- **Exercise While Watching TV**: Consider adding light exercises—like stretching, lunges, or core work—while watching your favorite show in the evening. These small additions make it easy to incorporate fitness into activities you already enjoy.

Pairing workouts with everyday activities helps make fitness feel more integrated, reducing the need for motivation and increasing consistency.

Establish Reminders to Reduce the Chance of Skipping Sessions

Life can get busy, and it's easy to forget or put off workouts. Setting reminders keeps fitness top of mind, ensuring you don't overlook your goals amidst daily responsibilities. Small nudges make a big difference in staying on track.

- **Set Digital Reminders**: Use your phone or a fitness app to schedule reminders. A daily notification can help keep you accountable, even if it's just a gentle nudge to get moving. For example, a reminder to "Stretch and hydrate!" every morning can reinforce your routine.

- **Create Visible Cues**: Place fitness equipment like resistance bands or a yoga mat somewhere visible to remind you of your commitment. Just seeing your equipment out can be a cue to get started.

- **Use Habit Trackers**: Whether it's a fitness app or a calendar, tracking completed workouts helps reinforce consistency. Marking off each day you complete your workout provides a sense of accomplishment and helps you visually track your progress.

Reminders and cues reduce the likelihood of skipping a workout, keeping you focused on your goals and strengthening your routine over time.

Building a routine that fits your life empowers you to stay consistent with ease and enjoyment. By identifying the best workout times, integrating exercise into your daily activities, and setting helpful reminders, you establish a sustainable routine that feels like a natural part of your day. These practices create a supportive environment for your fitness journey, making it easier to stick to your routine and build lasting habits.

Creating Accountability When Working Out Solo

Staying accountable is one of the biggest challenges when working out alone. Without a gym buddy or class instructor, it's easy to let motivation slip. However, there are powerful ways to create accountability on your own, making sure you stay on track with your fitness goals. By using digital tools, sharing your goals with trusted people, and setting up regular check-ins, you can cultivate a strong support system—even when exercising solo.

Use Apps or Trackers for Virtual Accountability

Fitness apps and trackers are excellent tools for accountability, allowing you to monitor your progress, set reminders, and keep a record of each workout. These digital companions help you stay committed by offering structured plans and progress tracking.

- **Choose a Comprehensive Fitness App**: Apps like MyFitnessPal, Strava, or Fitbit can be customized to your fitness goals, from tracking calorie intake to monitoring daily steps and workouts. Many of these apps provide reminders and weekly progress reports, helping you visualize your commitment.

- **Join Virtual Challenges**: Some apps and fitness communities offer monthly challenges or streak goals. Participating in these adds an extra layer of motivation, as you push yourself to complete a set number of workouts or achieve specific milestones.

- **Set Daily Reminders**: Schedule reminders in your app to keep workouts top of mind. Notifications serve as gentle nudges, reducing the likelihood of missed sessions and keeping you accountable on days when motivation is low.

Using digital trackers provides a structured way to monitor your journey, and seeing your progress builds momentum that fuels ongoing consistency.

Consider Sharing Goals with a Friend or Family Member

Sharing your fitness goals with someone close to you adds a valuable layer of accountability. When you communicate your plans to someone who supports your efforts, you're more likely to follow through and stay motivated.

- **Select a Supportive Partner**: Whether it's a friend, partner, or family member, choose someone who understands your goals and can offer positive encouragement. Having someone check in on your progress or simply cheer you on adds a sense of commitment.

- **Schedule Updates or Progress Talks**: Plan a weekly or monthly update session to discuss your progress. Knowing that someone else is tracking your journey can help you stay on course, even on challenging days.

- **Invite Feedback**: If your accountability partner has their own fitness experience, ask for advice or insights. Sometimes, an outside perspective can be incredibly valuable in helping you stay motivated or find new strategies.

Sharing your goals creates a social support system that reinforces your commitment to fitness, giving you someone to celebrate with when you reach milestones and to keep you going when motivation wanes.

Set Up Check-Ins to Stay on Track with Your Fitness Plan

Regular check-ins allow you to reflect on your progress, reassess your goals, and adjust your plans as needed. These moments of self-assessment help you stay connected to your intentions and see how far you've come, encouraging you to keep moving forward.

- **Plan Weekly or Monthly Check-Ins**: Schedule a set day each week or month to review your progress and track any changes. During this time, ask yourself questions like: "What went well?" "What challenges did I face?" "What adjustments do I need?"

- **Use a Journal or Tracking Tool**: Keep a fitness journal or use an app to document these check-ins. Recording your thoughts and observations provides a clear record of your journey, making it easier to identify patterns and celebrate achievements.

- **Adjust Goals as Needed**: Your fitness goals may shift as you progress, so use these check-ins to reevaluate what you're aiming for. Perhaps you want to add more cardio or start focusing on flexibility. Adjusting your goals keeps your routine fresh and aligned with your current abilities and interests.

Consistent check-ins provide valuable feedback on your progress, helping you stay committed to your fitness journey and giving you a sense of accomplishment along the way.

Creating accountability when working out solo doesn't have to be challenging. By using apps, sharing your goals with a supportive partner, and scheduling regular check-ins, you create a structured support system that keeps you motivated and on track. These strategies make your journey feel more engaging and rewarding, providing the encouragement you need to stick with your fitness routine, one workout at a time.

Techniques to Boost Motivation

Staying motivated can be another big challenge in your solo fitness journey. Without a gym environment or workout partner to push you, it's essential to find ways to keep yourself energized and committed. By setting short-term challenges, varying your routines, and reminding yourself of your "why," you can build lasting motivation that propels you forward.

Set Short-Term Challenges to Keep Things Exciting

Short-term challenges are a fantastic way to keep your fitness journey engaging. These goals bring a sense of urgency and accomplishment, helping you stay focused and eager to hit each target.

- **Try Weekly or Monthly Goals**: For example, challenge yourself to master a specific exercise, like doing a certain number of push-ups or increasing the duration of a plank. Short-term challenges like these provide quick wins and a steady sense of progress.

- **Experiment with Fitness Benchmarks**: Test your limits with metrics like time trials or endurance tests, such as "How many squats can I do in one minute?" or "Can I shave a minute off my usual run time?" Reaching these benchmarks is exciting and offers concrete proof of your improvement.

- **Reward Yourself**: Each time you complete a challenge, celebrate in a small way. This might mean treating yourself to a favorite snack, a new fitness accessory, or simply acknowledging your hard work. Rewards make challenges feel worthwhile and reinforce positive behavior.

Short-term challenges give you regular boosts of motivation, making it easier to stay on track and look forward to each workout.

Mix Up Routines with New Moves or Workouts

Variety is key to staying mentally engaged and physically challenged. A stagnant routine can lead to boredom, which makes it easier to skip workouts. By mixing things up, you keep your workouts fresh, enjoyable, and effective.

- **Introduce New Exercises Weekly**: Adding one or two new exercises, like kettlebell swings or mountain climbers, each week helps keep your routine interesting. New moves can target different muscle groups or work familiar ones in different ways, keeping your body challenged.

- **Try Different Workout Styles**: Explore different types of workouts, such as yoga, HIIT, or Pilates, to broaden your skill set and add variety. Not only does this introduce new challenges, but it also ensures a more well-rounded fitness regimen, with a balance of strength, endurance, and flexibility.

- **Use Music or Video Workouts**: Music has a powerful impact on motivation, so put together playlists that match your workout intensity. Alternatively, follow along with video workouts—having an instructor lead you through can provide structure and motivation, even from home.

Changing your routine regularly combats boredom, re-engages your focus, and helps you discover new types of exercise that you enjoy.

Reflect on the Reasons Behind Your Fitness Journey

Taking time to reflect on the deeper reasons behind your fitness goals gives meaning to your efforts and reinforces your commitment to self-improvement. When you connect with your "why," you create a source of motivation that runs deeper than external rewards.

- **Journal About Your Motivation**: Write down why you started your fitness journey in the first place, whether it's to feel healthier, gain confidence, or have more energy for your family. Keep this journal nearby, and revisit your entries whenever motivation dips.

- **Create a Vision Board**: A visual reminder of your goals can be powerful. Fill it with quotes, images, or personal milestones that inspire you. For example, place photos that represent your goals, like feeling energetic enough to play with your kids or reaching a specific fitness milestone.

- **Reflect Regularly**: Set aside a few minutes each week to remind yourself why you're working out. This reflection time can renew your motivation, especially on days when working out feels like a struggle.

Understanding your reasons for working out goes beyond any individual workout, connecting your actions to a greater purpose and keeping you driven through ups and downs.

By setting short-term challenges, varying your workouts, and reflecting on your motivations, you can maintain a high level of motivation on your fitness journey. These techniques not only keep things exciting but also remind you of the powerful reasons behind your commitment to fitness. As you move forward, remember that motivation isn't a constant; it's something you can actively cultivate through intentional choices and routines.

Overcoming Plateaus and Staying Engaged

Recognizing Signs of a Plateau

In any fitness journey, encountering a plateau is a common experience. Plateaus can be frustrating, but recognizing the signs early on allows you to adjust your approach and push past them. Knowing when your workouts have become too routine, spotting signs of burnout, and monitoring your progress will help you stay energized and on track toward your goals.

Note When Workouts Feel Routine or Progress Stalls

One of the first signs of a plateau is when your workouts start to feel predictable and uninspired. If your body becomes too accustomed to a set routine, the initial physical gains will eventually slow, and your motivation may follow suit.

- **Assess Your Routine**: If you've been doing the same exercises, reps, or duration for weeks without change, it might be time to switch things up. Small tweaks, like adding more weight or trying new exercises, can reignite your progress and re engage your muscles.

- **Look for Physical Stagnation**: Pay attention to whether you're still hitting new milestones. If your strength, endurance, or flexibility has stopped improving, this could signal that your body is no longer being challenged. To combat this, try incorporating progressive overload, such as adding more reps or resistance.

- **Keep Things Dynamic**: Experiment with different workout types or combinations to keep your body and mind engaged. Introducing new challenges ensures continuous progress and prevents your fitness routine from feeling stale.

Recognizing when workouts feel too predictable or progress stalls helps you identify when your body is craving change, a crucial step in overcoming a plateau.

Watch for Signs of Burnout or Loss of Motivation

Plateaus aren't just physical; they can also affect your mental state. Feelings of burnout or a noticeable dip in motivation can often signal that you're pushing too hard without adequate variation or recovery.

Listen to Your Mind and Body: If you're feeling unusually tired, unmotivated, or uninterested in your workouts, you may need a break or change in your routine. Burnout can be as detrimental to progress as physical stagnation, so don't overlook these signs. Incorporate Recovery and Rest: A plateau can sometimes be the body's way of asking for rest. Include active recovery days, stretching sessions, or even a short break to recharge both mentally and physically. Set New Goals: Loss of motivation can also occur when you're no longer excited about your current goals. Revisit your fitness goals and consider updating them to something that sparks renewed enthusiasm, like mastering a new exercise or hitting a different fitness benchmark.

Noticing signs of burnout or a dip in motivation allows you to take proactive steps, whether through rest, goal-setting, or adjusting your routine, to reignite your drive.

Monitor Workout Results to Detect Slowed Progress

Tracking your results over time is essential to recognizing when progress has slowed. Monitoring your performance helps you notice even subtle shifts, giving you an early warning when you may be reaching a plateau.

- **Record Key Metrics**: Keep track of relevant measurements like strength gains, endurance improvements, or flexibility. Even small data points, like being able to lift slightly more weight or complete an extra rep, indicate forward movement.

- **Take Note of Performance Changes**: If you consistently feel you're putting in the same effort but aren't achieving new results, it's worth reassessing your approach. A plateau often means your body has adapted to your current regimen, signaling it's time to intensify or diversify.

- **Reflect on Progress Regularly**: Schedule a monthly check-in to review your progress notes, whether they're in a fitness app, journal, or spreadsheet. Tracking your journey over time gives you a clear picture of when and where adjustments are needed.

Monitoring your progress provides tangible feedback, allowing you to catch and respond to plateaus quickly to stay on the path to achieving your fitness goals.

Recognizing signs of a plateau—whether physical, mental, or through slowed progress—enables you to make timely adjustments and avoid unnecessary frustration. By keeping your workouts dynamic, watching for burnout, and tracking your results, you can stay mindful of plateaus and work through them with ease and confidence. Each plateau you overcome brings you closer to the strength, resilience, and fitness goals you set out to achieve.

Introducing Variations to Stay Challenged

In any fitness journey, keeping things fresh and challenging is essential for both mental engagement and physical progress. By incorporating new movements, adjusting rep schemes, or adding equipment, you prevent your workouts from becoming predictable and keep your body adapting. Experimenting with different types of intensity, like supersets and dropsets, can also give your routine the boost it needs to keep challenging you.

Explore New Movements, Rep Schemes, or Workout Types

Adding variety to your exercises and rep schemes can make a significant difference in how effective and engaging your workouts feel. New moves or workout types target muscles differently, helping you break through plateaus and improve overall fitness.

- **Try Different Exercises**: Swap out standard moves with variations, such as trying sumo squats instead of regular squats, or experimenting with wide push-ups to engage different muscle fibers. These changes not only keep your workouts exciting but also work your body in new ways.

- **Vary Your Rep Schemes**: Instead of sticking to the same sets and reps, mix it up by incorporating pyramid sets (starting with low reps, building up, and then reducing reps) or working in time-based intervals instead of rep counts. These adjustments create different demands on your muscles and encourage greater strength and endurance gains.

- **Explore New Workout Styles**: Occasionally switch up your regular routine with different styles like circuit training, yoga, or Pilates. Cross-training with diverse exercises offers a refreshing change and ensures a balanced workout across strength, flexibility, and cardio.

New movements and rep schemes challenge your body to adapt to unfamiliar demands, keeping you engaged and constantly progressing toward your goals.

Add Equipment If Possible to Bring Variety

If you're working out with limited equipment, adding new items—even minimal ones—can provide a wealth of new exercise options. Small investments like resistance bands or a set of dumbbells can bring variety and extra resistance, keeping your muscles from getting too comfortable.

- **Introduce Resistance Bands**: These are excellent for home workouts due to their versatility and affordability. Bands can add resistance to familiar moves like squats or lunges, making each repetition more challenging and effective.

- **Experiment with Dumbbells or Kettlebells**: Adding

weights allows for greater muscle engagement, especially for exercises like deadlifts, shoulder presses, and lunges. Adjustable dumbbells or kettlebells can be especially valuable for a range of resistance options.

Consider Bodyweight Accessories: Even simple additions like a pull-up bar or stability ball can open up new exercises for building strength and stability, further expanding your options without taking up much space.

Adding equipment brings fresh challenges and helps you break through plateaus, keeping your routine versatile and your progress consistent.

Experiment with Intensity (e.g., Supersetting, Dropsets)

Increasing the intensity of your workouts is an effective way to stay challenged without needing more equipment or time. Supersets, dropsets, and other intensity techniques push your muscles to work harder, helping you make gains in strength and endurance.

- **Try Supersets for Efficiency and Intensity**: Supersets involve performing two exercises back-to-back with minimal rest. For example, combining push-ups with tricep dips targets different muscle groups quickly, keeping your heart rate up and challenging your muscles with minimal downtime.

- **Incorporate Dropsets for Extra Burn**I: In a dropset, you start with a heavy weight and decrease it after each set, continuing until your muscles reach fatigue. Dropsets are great for exercises like bicep curls or shoulder presses, where you can gradually reduce resistance and keep pushing beyond your initial limit.

- **Play with Tempo and Rest Periods**: Adjusting the pace of your reps or reducing rest between sets can create a new kind of challenge. For instance, slower eccentric (lowering) movements increase time under tension, adding intensity without extra weight.

Intensity techniques like supersets and dropsets ensure that even familiar exercises feel challenging, helping you make progress and preventing your body from settling into a routine.

Incorporating variety through new movements, equipment, and intensity techniques brings excitement and challenge to your workouts, helping you stay motivated and avoid plateaus. By regularly exploring these options, you keep your routine dynamic, ensuring continuous improvement and a more enjoyable fitness journey. As you experiment with different variations, you'll find new ways to push your limits and stay fully engaged in your solo workouts.

Finding Inspiration in Personal Growth

One of the most powerful motivators in a solo fitness journey is the personal growth you experience along the way. When you shift your focus from external results to internal progress, each workout becomes a meaningful step forward. Reflecting on your achievements, tracking mental health benefits, and embracing each session as part of a healthier lifestyle brings long-lasting inspiration that keeps you moving forward.

Reflect on Past Achievements and Improvements

Looking back on how far you've come is a great way to maintain motivation and find inspiration. Celebrating the milestones you've already reached—no matter how small—reminds you of your dedication and progress, reinforcing the power of consistency.

- **Acknowledge Physical Progress**: Whether it's lifting heavier weights, mastering a new movement, or simply building up your endurance, each of these achievements reflects your commitment and resilience. Take time to recognize these wins as proof of your ability to grow and improve.

- **Recognize Skill Development**: Beyond physical gains, you've likely developed skills, improved form, or gained knowledge about exercise techniques. Each skill you gain enriches your fitness journey, empowering you to take on new challenges.

- **Capture Milestones in a Journal**: Writing down your successes allows you to revisit them anytime you need a confidence boost. Reflecting on past accomplishments keeps your vision forward-focused, giving you a renewed sense of purpose and drive for each session.

Reflecting on past achievements helps you stay connected to your progress, reminding you that each step has built a foundation for where you are now and where you're heading next.

Keep Track of Mental Health Benefits Along with Physical Progress

Physical gains are just part of the picture. Regular exercise provides substantial mental and emotional benefits that often go unnoticed but play a crucial role in keeping you inspired and balanced. Recognizing these benefits reminds you that your efforts have a positive impact on both body and mind.

- **Observe Emotional Shifts**: Pay attention to improvements in mood, focus, and stress levels after workouts. Exercise is a proven mood-booster, thanks to the endorphins and serotonin it releases. Tracking these benefits helps you connect your physical routine with a healthier, happier mindset.

- **Measure Confidence Gains**: Solo workouts require self-motivation, and achieving even small goals on your own builds self-confidence. Notice how meeting challenges in fitness translates to feeling more capable in other areas of life.

- **Note Energy and Productivity Levels**: Consistent exercise often leads to increased energy and productivity. Logging how energized you feel post-workout highlights the broader lifestyle benefits of staying active.

Recording these mental health benefits along with your physical progress reminds you that every workout improves not only your strength but also your well-being, motivation, and overall quality of life.

Embrace Each Workout as a Step Toward a Healthier Lifestyle

Each workout is an investment in your long-term health and happiness. By viewing every session as a step forward, you begin to see exercise as a daily commitment to yourself—a way of living that values health, strength, and self-care.

- **See Progress Beyond the Gym**: Every positive habit you build through your workouts reinforces a lifestyle focused on well-being. From healthy eating to better sleep, the impact of regular exercise extends far beyond your fitness routine.

- **Find Joy in the Process, Not Just the Outcome**: Fitness isn't just about reaching a goal; it's about learning to love the journey.

Each workout becomes meaningful when you approach it as an act of self-care, one that contributes to your physical and mental resilience.

- **Create a Long-Term Vision**: Visualize how your commitment to fitness supports the person you want to become, both now and in the future. This vision gives purpose to every workout, helping you appreciate each moment as a valuable part of your growth.

By embracing each workout as a step toward a healthier lifestyle, you develop a strong sense of purpose in your fitness journey. Every session contributes to a foundation of health and resilience, inspiring you to stay committed and excited for what's to come.

Finding inspiration in personal growth is about celebrating every step—physical and mental—that you take toward a better version of yourself. When you appreciate the journey, track both physical and mental progress, and embrace each workout as part of your evolving lifestyle, you create a lasting source of motivation that will carry you forward, no matter the challenges you face.

Chapter 4: Creating Long-Term Success Beyond the Gym

Developing a Sustainable, Lifelong Approach

Focusing on Health Beyond Aesthetic

When fitness becomes about more than just appearance, it transforms into a deeply fulfilling and sustainable journey. Shifting your focus from aesthetic goals to goals rooted in strength, energy, and overall well-being helps you stay inspired by the true value of exercise: feeling better each day, building resilience, and enhancing your quality of life. This perspective empowers you to embrace fitness as a long-term commitment to yourself, not just as a means to reach a physical ideal.

Set Goals Related to Strength, Energy, and Well-Being

Focusing on functional and personal goals makes each workout purposeful and rewarding. Goals that emphasize strength, energy, and mental health create a balanced approach that supports your whole self.

- **Prioritize Strength and Stamina**: Training to improve your strength, endurance, and mobility allows you to see progress beyond visual changes. Each new personal best—whether it's lifting more weight, completing more reps, or running longer—represents real, tangible progress that's grounded in health and ability.

- **Measure Energy Levels and Daily Performance**: Pay attention to how you feel after workouts and throughout the day. Increased energy, better sleep, and improved focus are powerful indicators of a healthy, balanced body. Set goals around these benefits to stay motivated by how exercise positively impacts your daily life.

- **Nurture Mental Health and Resilience**: Physical exercise has profound effects on mental health. Setting goals related to stress relief, mental clarity, or emotional stability reminds you that each session supports a healthier, happier mind.

By focusing on strength, energy, and well-being, you create goals that are meaningful, sustainable, and empowering, making your fitness journey feel rewarding from the inside out.

Avoid Comparing Yourself to Others or Focusing Solely on Looks

One of the most liberating aspects of solo fitness is that it's just you against your own goals. Without external pressure or the comparison trap of the gym, you can define success on your own terms and focus solely on personal growth. Avoiding comparisons and aesthetic fixation helps you maintain a healthy, positive mindset.

- **Recognize Your Unique Journey**: Fitness is deeply personal, and everyone's journey is unique. Avoid comparing your progress or appearance to others by remembering that your goals are centered on what's best for you. Your journey, your pace, and your achievements are yours alone.

- **Prioritize Inner Strength Over Outer Appearances:** While aesthetic changes can be a motivating byproduct of exercise, it's important not to let looks overshadow the health benefits. By prioritizing how you feel, rather than how you look, you create a stronger bond with the process itself, helping you stay committed long-term.

- **Celebrate Non-Physical Wins**: Progress can be seen in how much better you feel each day, how much stronger or more capable you become, or how many new skills you master. By celebrating these achievements, you reinforce your commitment to health and happiness rather than surface-level results.

Letting go of comparisons and focusing on internal goals creates a healthy, positive relationship with fitness, one where your motivation comes from within, unaffected by external expectations.

Embrace Fitness as a Means to Feel Better Daily

When exercise is about feeling better in your daily life, it becomes a source of joy and self-care rather than a chore. Fitness becomes part of a lifestyle that prioritizes your well-being, enhancing everything from your mood to your resilience.

- **Look Forward to Each Workout as a Self-Care Ritual**: Treat each session as a gift to yourself, a chance to reconnect with your body, recharge your mind, and release stress. When exercise becomes a ritual of self-care, it's easier to stay consistent and committed.

- **Appreciate Daily Benefits Beyond the Gym**: Fitness impacts every part of your life—from increased energy to improved mental clarity. Notice how each workout translates into feeling more alive, empowered, and capable in your daily activities. These small, everyday wins remind you of the value in each session.

- **Align Your Goals with Long-Term Health**: Seeing fitness as a lifelong journey makes it easier to remain motivated and adaptable, even when progress seems slow. When each workout is part of a commitment to long-term health, your focus shifts to the positive impact exercise has on your body and mind over time.

By focusing on health beyond aesthetics, you cultivate a deep appreciation for what fitness can do for your life. When strength, energy, and well-being become your markers of progress, fitness becomes a sustainable, positive part of who you are. Embracing this mindset keeps you motivated for the right reasons, helping you stay consistent and dedicated to your goals, day after day, with a focus on feeling your best from the inside out.

Finding Joy in the Process of Fitness

One of the greatest rewards of a solo fitness journey is the ability to shape it around what truly brings you joy and fulfillment. When you focus on the aspects you genuinely enjoy, exercise becomes more than a task—it transforms into a form of self-expression, mindfulness, and even relaxation. By making space for enjoyment, flexibility, and mental well-being, you create a routine that feels both refreshing and motivating, making it easier to stay consistent for the long term.

Identify Movements and Exercises You Genuinely Enjoy

Fitness should never feel like a chore. Finding exercises you love transforms each workout into something to look forward to and makes it easier to stay consistent. When you enjoy the movements, your motivation naturally increases, and working out becomes a fun, energizing part of your routine.

- **Experiment to Discover What Clicks**: Try out different styles—strength training, bodyweight circuits, yoga, or dance workouts. By exploring various types of exercise, you can discover what truly resonates with you and build routines that include movements that excite you.

- **Incorporate Activities that Feel Natural**: Choosing exercises that align with your natural abilities or interests can make fitness feel less forced and more enjoyable. For instance, if you love rhythm, add in some aerobic or dance-style exercises. If you prefer a slow, controlled pace, focus on strength moves or flexibility work.

- **Make It Personal**: Your solo fitness journey is entirely yours, which means there's no pressure to follow what others are doing. Whether you're jumping into cardio circuits or practicing calming yoga flows, pick the activities that feel right for you, enhancing the joy you find in each session.

Use Solo Workouts as a Mental Reset or Mindfulness Practice

Solo workouts can provide much more than physical benefits—they offer a chance to reset your mind and find peace within your day. Approaching fitness as a mindfulness practice can make it feel like a break from stress rather than an obligation, encouraging you to be fully present in each movement.

- **Embrace the Mind-Body Connection**: Pay close attention to your breathing, posture, and the sensation of each movement. This focus not only improves your form and results but also brings a sense of calm and mindfulness, transforming exercise into a moving meditation.

- **Use Workouts to Clear Your Mind**: Solo workouts provide a peaceful space for clearing your mind and re-centering yourself. Letting go of daily stress and immersing yourself in each exercise gives you a mental break that can refresh and recharge your energy.

- **Celebrate the Emotional Benefits**: Recognize how much better you feel mentally and emotionally after a workout. This awareness reinforces exercise as a valuable tool for emotional well-being, making you look forward to each session as a mental escape or personal recharge.

Allow for Occasional Flexibility in Routines to Keep Interest

Routines are important for consistency, but a little flexibility keeps your fitness journey exciting and fresh. Giving yourself permission to change things up helps prevent boredom, keeps you mentally engaged, and allows you to adapt based on your energy, mood, or goals.

- **Switch Things Up When Needed**: If a workout feels repetitive or uninspiring, try introducing new movements, altering the order of exercises, or experimenting with different intensities. This variety keeps you curious and prevents the routine from feeling stagnant.

- **Listen to Your Body and Mind**: Some days, you may feel energetic and ready for a challenge; on others, you might benefit from a slower, more restorative workout. Allowing yourself to modify your plans based on what you need that day keeps your routine sustainable and enjoyable.

- **Embrace the Freedom of Solo Workouts**: The beauty of working out alone is that you can set your own pace and adjust as you go. Without the constraints of a class schedule or gym setup, you're free to explore, modify, and tailor your routine to keep it both effective and exciting.

Finding joy in the process of fitness is about more than the physical—it's about feeling good mentally, staying engaged, and making each workout a meaningful part of your life. When you choose exercises that make you happy, use workouts as a mental reset, and add flexibility to keep things interesting, you create a fitness journey that's enjoyable, fulfilling, and truly yours. Embracing this joyful approach to fitness ensures that each session becomes a positive, uplifting experience, making it easier to stay consistent and inspired along the way.

Building Lasting Habits

The secret to a sustainable fitness journey lies in transforming workouts into a regular, non-negotiable part of your daily life. When fitness becomes a habit rather than an occasional activity, you cultivate a foundation of discipline and self-care that supports long-term growth. By committing to a consistent schedule, embracing discipline, and regularly reflecting on what works best for you, you can build a routine that feels natural, rewarding, and resilient.

Make Workouts a Non-Negotiable Part of Daily Life

One of the most effective ways to ensure consistency in fitness is to treat it as an essential part of your routine, just like any other important daily activity. When exercise becomes something you do out of habit, it no longer relies on temporary motivation or willpower—it's simply part of who you are and what you do.

- **Schedule It Like an Appointmen**t: Set aside specific times each day or week that are solely dedicated to your workout. By treating this time as a personal commitment, you reinforce the idea that fitness is essential to your routine, making it less likely to be skipped.

- **Attach Meaning to Your Routine**: Remind yourself why exercise is important to you—whether for health, energy, mental clarity, or self-confidence. This personal meaning reinforces the idea that workouts aren't optional; they're a valuable investment in your well-being.

- **Embrace Exercise as a Form of Self-Respect**: Making workouts non-negotiable sends a powerful message that you value your health and are dedicated to your goals. When you view each session as an act of self-respect, it becomes easier to follow through consistently.

Maintain Discipline by Sticking to a Consistent Schedule

Discipline is the key to transforming any new activity into a lasting habit. By sticking to a consistent workout schedule, you train your mind and body to expect and prepare for this routine, making it feel increasingly natural over time.

- **Create a Routine That Fits Your Life**: Set realistic and achievable workout days and times, based on your lifestyle. For instance, if you're more energized in the morning, aim to work out then. Consistency is about fitting workouts into your life in a way that feels manageable and sustainable.

- **Establish Positive Cues and Reminders**: Use reminders, whether through alarms, sticky notes, or apps, to help you remember and anticipate your workout times. Setting visual or digital cues reinforces your routine, making it easier to stay on track each day.

- **Honor Your Schedule, Even on Tough Days**: Some days will be harder than others, but showing up, even for a shorter or modified session, builds mental strength. Consistency breeds discipline, and each time you follow through, you reinforce the habit, making future workouts feel easier to commit to.

Reflect Regularly to Understand and Sustain What Works Best

Building a lasting fitness habit also requires periodic reflection to assess what is or isn't working for you. Taking time to evaluate your routines helps you make adjustments, stay aligned with your goals, and sustain motivation over the long term.

- **Track Progress and Patterns**: Keep a simple log of your workouts and how they make you feel. Over time, you'll notice patterns—such as the times you feel most motivated or the types of exercises you enjoy most—that help you optimize your schedule.

- **Celebrate Small Wins**: Regularly reflecting on your achievements, big or small, reinforces your commitment and boosts your motivation. Celebrating these moments reminds you of the progress you're making, encouraging you to stay consistent.

- **Adjust and Adapt as Needed**: Habits that work today may need to shift as life changes or as your fitness levels improve. By reflecting on what keeps you engaged and what may need tweaking, you can adapt your approach, ensuring your routine remains enjoyable and effective.

By making workouts a non-negotiable part of daily life, maintaining discipline with a consistent schedule, and reflecting regularly on what works best, you build a strong foundation for lasting fitness habits. This commitment to routine not only helps you achieve physical goals but also empowers you to cultivate resilience, self-discipline, and personal growth. With these practices in place, fitness becomes a fulfilling, enduring part of who you are, supporting you in living your healthiest, happiest life.

Preventing Injuries and Staying Safe at Home

Warm-up and Cool-down Essentials

A well-rounded fitness routine doesn't just include the main workout—it begins with a thoughtful warm-up and ends with a mindful cooldown. These essential components help you maximize the benefits of your workouts while reducing the risk of injury, enhancing flexibility, and promoting overall recovery. By giving proper attention to warm-up and cool-down phases, you set yourself up for a safer, more effective, and enjoyable fitness journey.

Begin with Dynamic Stretches to Prepare Muscles

Dynamic stretches are an ideal way to start any workout, as they engage your muscles and elevate your heart rate, preparing your body for movement. Unlike static stretches, which involve holding a position, dynamic stretches keep you moving, promoting blood flow to the muscles you'll be using.

- **Activate Key Muscle Groups**: Choose stretches that target the areas you plan to work on, such as leg swings before a lower-body session or arm circles before an upper-body workout. This targeted approach ensures that your muscles are primed and ready.

- **Increase Joint Mobility**: Dynamic stretches, like lunges with a twist or torso rotations, also increase the range of motion in your joints, helping to enhance flexibility and prevent stiffness during your workout.

- **Gradually Boost Your Heart Rate**: By slowly raising your heart rate through movements like high knees or arm swings, you allow your cardiovascular system to adjust, reducing strain and preparing your body for more intense activity.

Focus on Breathing and Proper Form Throughout the Session

Breath and form are two foundational aspects of any workout. Paying attention to both not only supports effective movement but also enhances endurance, stability, and focus throughout each session.

- **Practice Controlled Breathing**: Developing a breathing rhythm that aligns with your movement can improve oxygen flow and help prevent fatigue. For example, inhale during easier parts of the movement and exhale during exertion, such as when lifting or pushing.

- **Prioritize Form Over Speed or Intensity**: Quality movement leads to better results and lowers injury risk. Take time to focus on your posture, alignment, and control. For instance, when squatting, ensure that your knees track over your toes and that your back remains straight.

- **Stay Mindful of Each Movement**: Concentrating on each movement helps you remain present and enhances the mind-muscle connection, maximizing the effectiveness of each exercise and supporting overall stability.

Use Cooldown Stretches to Aid in Recovery and Flexibility

Ending with a cooldown phase helps your body return to a resting state while promoting recovery and flexibility. This phase is crucial for preventing muscle tightness, reducing soreness, and ensuring that your body is ready for the next workout.

- **Incorporate Static Stretches for Key Muscles**: Unlike the dynamic stretches in your warm-up, cooldown stretches should be static, meaning you hold each stretch for 15-30 seconds. Target the muscles you worked on during the session, allowing each to relax and lengthen.

- **Relax with Deep Breathing**: Slow, deep breaths during your cooldown help to calm your nervous system and enhance relaxation. This mindful breathing allows you to wind down, releasing any tension in your muscles and promoting a sense of calm.

- **Encourage Flexibility and Prevent Stiffness**: Regularly incorporating cooldown stretches, like hamstring or shoulder stretches, not only helps with flexibility but also prevents post-workout stiffness. This added mobility supports a wider range of motion over time, enhancing your future workouts.

By integrating a thoughtful warm-up and cooldown into every session, you ensure that your body is fully prepared for each workout and supported in its recovery. These essential components not only make your workouts safer but also enhance their overall quality, allowing you to perform better and feel stronger. Starting with dynamic stretches, focusing on breathing and form, and ending with cooldown stretches are simple but powerful steps that elevate your fitness routine and help sustain long-term progress.

Proper Form and Technique for Solo Exercisers

When working out alone, maintaining proper form and technique is essential for effective, safe training. Without a trainer or spotter, solo exercisers need to be extra mindful of their movements to prevent injury and maximize gains. By recognizing the difference between muscle fatigue and injury pain, using tools to self-correct form, and avoiding excessive weights, you can create a workout environment that prioritizes safety and promotes lasting progress.

Differentiate Between Muscle Fatigue and Injury Pain

One of the most critical aspects of training solo is understanding the signals your body sends. Knowing when to push through muscle fatigue and when to stop due to injury pain can prevent minor issues from turning into serious setbacks.

- **Understand Muscle Fatigue**: Muscle fatigue is a natural response to a challenging workout, often characterized by a "burning" sensation or general tiredness in the muscle. This type of discomfort is typically safe and even beneficial for building strength, as long as it doesn't cross into pain.

- **Recognize Signs of Injury Pain**: Unlike fatigue, injury pain is often sharp, sudden, or located in a joint rather than the muscle itself. If you feel a sharp, pinching sensation or experience joint discomfort, stop immediately and assess the area. Pushing through injury pain can lead to strains or other serious injuries.

- **Learn Your Limits**: Listen to your body, and understand that fatigue is a signal to rest, while pain is a cue to reevaluate. Over time, you'll develop a stronger sense of your body's signals, helping you distinguish between healthy exertion and signs of strain.

Use Mirrors or Video to Self-Correct Form if Needed

Maintaining proper form is essential for effective and safe solo workouts. Without a trainer to provide real-time feedback, mirrors or videos can be valuable tools for monitoring your alignment and technique.

Position a Mirror in Your Workout Space: A mirror provides instant visual feedback, allowing you to check your posture, alignment, and movement. If you notice any imbalance or misalignment, adjust immediately to ensure proper form. Record Yourself on Video: Filming yourself during exercises can be especially helpful for moves that require more precision, such as deadlifts or squats. Review the footage to identify areas for improvement, paying close attention to alignment and movement control. Focus on Specific Form Cues: Each exercise has key form cues—for example, keeping your knees over your toes during squats or maintaining a straight back in planks. Memorize these cues for each move, and check in with yourself during workouts to stay mindful of your technique.

Avoid Overloading Weight to Prevent Strain

While lifting heavier weights can be beneficial for building strength, overloading too quickly or with improper form can lead to strain or injury. Solo exercisers should prioritize control and form over heavy weights to build strength safely.

Prioritize Form Over Weight: It's tempting to push your limits with heavier weights, but the safest way to progress is to master each exercise with proper form first. By focusing on quality over quantity, you ensure that your movements are controlled, reducing the risk of strain.

Progress Gradually: Increase weight or resistance in small increments as you build strength. This gradual progression allows your muscles and joints to adapt, minimizing the risk of injury from sudden increases in load. Consider Alternative Intensity Techniques: If you want to challenge yourself without adding excessive weight, try other techniques like slowing down the tempo of your movements or adding additional reps. These methods build strength without the need to overload.

By understanding muscle fatigue versus injury pain, using mirrors or videos for self-correction, and avoiding excessive weight, solo exercisers can confidently maintain proper form and technique. These practices create a safe, effective workout environment that empowers you to stay injury-free while achieving your fitness goals. Each workout becomes an opportunity to refine your technique, deepen your body awareness, and make steady progress toward your strongest self.

Recognizing and Addressing Pain Signals

In any fitness journey, knowing how to interpret your body's signals is key to staying safe and progressing effectively. For solo exercisers, understanding the difference between normal muscle fatigue and injury-related pain is crucial, as you may not have a trainer or workout partner to help identify issues in real time. By learning to adjust or stop exercises at the first sign of discomfort and consulting professionals when necessary, you'll be able to continue training with confidence and minimize the risk of injury.

Differentiate Between Muscle Fatigue and Injury Pain

Recognizing the difference between muscle fatigue, which is a natural part of building strength, and pain that could indicate injury, is essential. Each type of sensation tells you something different about what's happening in your body.

Muscle Fatigue is Normal and Expected: Muscle fatigue typically feels like a burning or tired sensation in the muscle as it becomes more difficult to continue the movement. This type of discomfort is generally safe and can be expected when pushing your limits in a workout. Fatigue is a sign your muscles are working and adapting to the challenge. Injury Pain is Sharp or Sudden: Unlike fatigue, injury pain often feels sharp, localized, or sudden and may affect areas like joints or tendons. This type of pain is your body's way of signaling that something isn't right, so it's important to take it seriously. If you feel a sharp twinge or pinching sensation, especially in joints, it's best to stop the exercise. Develop Body Awareness Over Time: With experience, you'll get better at interpreting your body's responses to different movements. When in doubt, treat sharp or unexpected pain as a signal to pause and assess.

Adjust or Stop Exercises if Discomfort Arises

If discomfort arises during a workout, it's essential to listen to your body and make adjustments as needed. Small changes in form or modifying an exercise can sometimes alleviate discomfort, but knowing when to stop is equally important.

Try a Modification First: If a specific movement feels uncomfortable, you can try a modified version to see if it relieves the discomfort. For instance, if lunges cause knee strain, try adjusting your stance or reducing the range of motion. Sometimes, minor tweaks can make a big difference. Stop at the First Sign of Injury Pain: If the discomfort persists or worsens, it's best to stop the exercise completely. Continuing with pain can lead to further injury, so it's essential to prioritize safety over completing a set. Take a Rest Day if Needed: If you notice lingering discomfort after a workout, consider taking an additional rest day or focusing on a different area of your body. Allowing time for recovery can prevent minor strains from turning into more significant injuries.

Consider Consulting Professionals if Pain Persists

Persistent pain is a clear indication that your body may need extra support. Consulting a professional, whether it's a physical therapist, doctor, or certified trainer, can provide valuable insight and help you address the issue effectively.

- **Physical Therapists for Pain Management**: A physical therapist can assess your movement and provide personalized exercises to address any imbalances or weaknesses. They can also offer modifications for exercises that may be contributing to discomfort.

- **Trainers for Technique Refinement**: If pain persists in specific exercises, a certified trainer can help assess and correct your form, which may alleviate discomfort. Sometimes, even minor adjustments to posture or alignment can make a difference.

- **Seek Medical Advice for Severe or Ongoing Pain**S: If pain is intense or doesn't improve after rest, it's essential to see a healthcare provider to rule out serious injury. Early intervention can prevent issues from worsening and support long-term progress.

By learning to recognize and address pain signals, you equip yourself with the tools to train safely and effectively. Differentiating between muscle fatigue and pain, making adjustments or stopping when necessary, and consulting professionals as needed are all vital steps in a sustainable fitness journey. Listening to your body not only helps you avoid injury but also enhances your understanding of how to work with your body's needs, supporting a lifetime of healthy, injury-free training.

Maintaining Progress and Growing Over Time

Periodic Self-Assessments

Regular self-assessment is key to maintaining progress and enthusiasm on your fitness journey. Taking time every few months to review your goals, evaluate your progress, and add new challenges keeps your routine fresh and ensures that your efforts are aligned with your evolving aspirations. Periodic self-assessment not only keeps you on track but also allows for continuous growth, making your fitness routine adaptable and exciting.

Review Your Goals Every Few Months to Ensure Alignment

As life changes, so do our priorities and goals. Every few months, take a step back and assess whether your current fitness goals align with where you are and what you want to achieve. Maybe your initial focus was on building strength, but now you'd like to add more flexibility or endurance work. Checking in with yourself helps maintain a sense of purpose and ensures that your workouts contribute meaningfully to your broader lifestyle and health goals.

- **Adjust for Life Circumstances**: For instance, if you've had an increase in work or family commitments, consider setting more achievable short-term goals to avoid feeling overwhelmed. On the other hand, if you have more time to dedicate to fitness, this might be a good opportunity to increase your workout intensity or frequency.

Revisit Your "Why": Reflect on the reasons behind your fitness journey. Are you still motivated by the same goals, or has your focus shifted? Keeping your "why" front and center helps you stay connected to the deeper purpose behind your workouts.

Re-evaluate Fitness Goals as Progress is Made

When you reach a milestone or a fitness goal, it's an ideal time to revisit and set new targets. Re-evaluating goals as you progress prevents stagnation and encourages continuous improvement.

Celebrate Successes, Then Set New Objectives: Every time you achieve a goal—whether it's lifting a heavier weight, completing a challenging workout, or consistently following your routine—take a moment to recognize that accomplishment. Then, consider what's next. Perhaps you can add more reps, increase the intensity, or explore a different fitness focus like endurance or mobility. Adjust the Goal Post as Needed: Progress isn't always linear, so it's also okay to shift goals if your current ones feel too demanding or if circumstances change. Staying flexible with your goals allows you to adapt to your body's needs and stay motivated without feeling pressured.

Consider Adding New Challenges to Maintain Enthusiasm

Adding variety to your routine can be invigorating and help sustain long-term motivation. Trying new exercises, incorporating different fitness equipment, or experimenting with workout styles (like HIIT, Pilates, or strength training) are excellent ways to add excitement. Diversify Your Workout Styles: If you've been focusing primarily on strength, try a yoga or flexibility-focused session. If you love cardio, consider strength training for balance. This variety not only keeps things fresh but also challenges different muscle groups, contributing to a well-rounded fitness routine. Challenge Yourself in New Ways: New challenges could be as simple as increasing weights, trying a more advanced movement, or setting a new personal best. These periodic challenges keep the journey engaging, and the excitement of trying something new can rekindle enthusiasm for solo workouts.

Q1: How do I identify when my goals are no longer aligned with my current lifestyle or fitness needs?

A1: A helpful approach is to look for signs of waning motivation, frustration with progress, or even boredom with your routine. These are often indicators that it's time for a goal check-in. Ask yourself if what you're currently doing is fulfilling, achievable, and conducive to your lifestyle. If not, realigning with goals that better fit your current circumstances can reignite your enthusiasm and make each session more rewarding.

Q2: What are some ways to celebrate small fitness milestones in a meaningful way?

A2: Celebrating fitness milestones can be simple yet impactful. Treat yourself to a new piece of workout gear, try a fun fitness activity you've been curious about, or set a dedicated "recovery day" with a relaxing activity like a spa session or nature hike. These celebrations not only mark your achievements but also provide positive reinforcement, reminding you of the progress you've made and motivating you to continue.

Q3: How can I add new challenges without overwhelming myself or risking burnout?

A3: Gradual changes are key. Start by adding one new element at a time, like increasing the weight on a specific exercise or trying a new workout style once a week. Make sure to balance these challenges with rest and recovery days. This method keeps things exciting without overloading your routine, allowing your body and mind to adapt while still feeling motivated by the added variety.

Expanding Fitness Knowledge

Learning continuously is essential to maintaining progress and avoiding stagnation in your fitness journey. Expanding your fitness knowledge—whether through fresh workout ideas, understanding body mechanics, or staying updated on fitness principles—can keep your solo routine dynamic and effective. By committing to lifelong learning, you gain the skills and insights to tailor your workouts more effectively, prevent plateaus, and stay motivated with an ever-evolving approach to fitness.

Explore Resources for Fresh Workout Ideas and Fitness Tips

The world of fitness is constantly evolving, and exploring new resources is a great way to keep your workouts interesting and aligned with current best practices. Online platforms, fitness apps, social media, and books are all rich sources of inspiration and knowledge.

- **Try New Workout Styles**: Consider exploring workouts like high-intensity interval training (HIIT), resistance band circuits, or bodyweight-focused routines to diversify your skills. By experimenting with different types of workouts, you can discover new ways to challenge your body and break up the routine.

- **Stay Up-to-Date on Tips from Experts**: Following trainers or fitness influencers who specialize in home-based or solo workouts can provide practical advice and fresh ideas. Subscribing to newsletters, YouTube channels, or fitness blogs is also a great way to stay connected to the latest fitness insights and keep your sessions engaging.

Stay Informed About Body Mechanics and Fitness Principles

Understanding how the body works during exercise can enhance the effectiveness and safety of your workouts. Knowing about proper alignment, muscle engagement, and body mechanics helps you achieve better form, reduce injury risk, and maximize the benefits of each movement.

- **Focus on Functional Anatomy**: Familiarizing yourself with basic muscle groups and joint functions will give you a greater appreciation of how each exercise impacts your body. Learning about core stabilization, muscle activation, and mobility work can also enhance your workouts, especially when performing complex or compound movements.

- **Study Key Fitness Principles**: Concepts like progressive overload, muscle recovery, and flexibility are fundamental to effective training. By understanding these principles, you'll be better equipped to design well-rounded routines that incorporate strength, endurance, and flexibility in a balanced way. This knowledge allows you to optimize each workout and maintain consistent progress.

Keep Learning to Prevent Plateaus and Stay Motivated

Continuous learning helps prevent fitness plateaus, where progress seems to stall despite regular effort. Learning new techniques or incorporating recent findings from fitness science can introduce fresh challenges that stimulate growth and keep you motivated.

- **Look into Specialized Workouts**: If you find your workouts feeling repetitive or you notice a decrease in progress, learning about specialized techniques like plyometric training or circuit training can reinvigorate your routine. These methods offer unique challenges that keep your body adapting and evolving.

- **Read and Reflect Regularly**: Periodically reading fitness articles, watching instructional videos, or even listening to health-related podcasts can introduce you to the latest insights, helping you add effective variations to your solo workouts. Keeping up with new information helps you stay committed to your journey, as you continuously discover ways to grow.

By dedicating time to expand your fitness knowledge, you're empowering yourself to maintain a sustainable and enjoyable fitness journey. The more you learn, the more tools you'll have to create challenging, effective, and safe workouts that align with your goals. With each new piece of information, you're not only enhancing your fitness level but also reinforcing your commitment to lifelong wellness.

Preparing for New Fitness Challenges

Setting new fitness challenges adds excitement and purpose to your journey, keeping your motivation high and your routines dynamic. Whether it's working toward a personal milestone or setting longer-term objectives, preparing for new challenges can reignite your passion for solo workouts and drive continuous improvement.

Set New Goals Like Completing a Personal Milestone or Event

Setting specific, achievable goals that push your limits can help you stay motivated and focused. These can be as simple as increasing the number of push-ups you can do or as ambitious as completing a fitness event.

- **Define Your Milestone**: Choose a target that inspires you, such as achieving a certain number of reps, reaching a personal best for a particular exercise, or finishing a set routine without breaks. These goals give you something tangible to work toward and offer a sense of accomplishment when achieved.

- **Consider a Personal Fitness Event**: Even if you're working out solo, you can create your own "event." For example, you could plan a challenge to complete a set number of exercises within a time frame, or even aim for a "personal best" day where you test your endurance, strength, or flexibility. These self-designed events serve as exciting benchmarks and encourage growth in various areas of fitness.

Take on Longer-Term Objectives to Keep Things Exciting

Once you've reached short-term goals, setting longer-term objectives can help you maintain momentum and enthusiasm. These broader goals might span months or even a year, giving you a reason to stay committed over time.

- **Plan for Consistent Growth**: Longer-term goals like improving overall flexibility, building muscle definition, or achieving a specific weight-lifting target give your fitness journey depth and structure. These goals encourage a steady, sustainable pace of progress and keep you engaged without the pressure of immediate results.

- **Break Down Large Goals into Smaller Steps**: For example, if your objective is to improve your endurance, create smaller milestones, like gradually increasing the length of each cardio session. Each mini-goal serves as a stepping stone toward your bigger objective and keeps you encouraged by visible, incremental progress.

Embrace the Journey of Continuous Improvement

Adopting a mindset of lifelong fitness means embracing the idea of continuous improvement. Instead of focusing solely on end goals, enjoy each step forward, knowing that fitness is an ongoing journey with room for growth at every level.

- **Recognize Small Wins**: Each workout and every small improvement contributes to your overall progress. Celebrate these wins, whether it's an extra rep, a new variation you've mastered, or a longer workout session. This approach not only builds confidence but also cultivates a positive attitude toward challenges.

- **Enjoy the Process of Self-Discovery**: As you face and overcome new fitness challenges, you'll learn more about your strengths, capabilities, and resilience. This journey allows you to connect more deeply with your body and mind, transforming fitness from a task into a fulfilling lifestyle.

Preparing for new challenges adds excitement to your solo fitness journey, ensuring there's always a fresh objective on the horizon. By setting specific goals, embracing long-term milestones, and celebrating each step of the process, you'll cultivate a sustainable, fulfilling approach to fitness that adapts to your evolving ambitions. With each new challenge, you reinforce the rewarding cycle of growth and accomplishment that makes solo fitness not just an activity but an empowering journey.

Conclusion: Your Journey to Lasting Solo Fitness

As we wrap up this journey together, let's revisit the core themes and insights we've covered. This book began with the promise of guiding you toward a fulfilling, effective solo fitness routine, showing that you don't need a crowded gym or expensive memberships to achieve your fitness goals. We looked at the benefits of working out on your own, embracing both peace and privacy while building strength and resilience.

We explored different workout options tailored for solo exercisers, from bodyweight routines to high-intensity intervals (HIIT), low-impact cardio, and strength exercises that don't require much space or equipment. We also examined how you can set SMART goals to keep your focus sharp and how to track and celebrate milestones to keep your motivation high. We talked about breaking through plateaus, adding variety to stay challenged, and ensuring that your workouts remain aligned with your evolving goals.

In the end, the aim of all this knowledge is to support you in building a routine that becomes a natural part of your life.

With insights into proper form, injury prevention, recovery, and self-assessment, you're equipped to stay consistent and adaptable as your fitness journey continues.

To everyone who has read through to the end, thank you. Writing this book was a labor of love, and knowing that it reached readers like you means everything. I hope these pages have empowered and inspired you to take charge of your fitness journey and to find joy and satisfaction in your solo workouts.

If you found this book valuable, I would be incredibly grateful if you could take a moment to leave a review on Amazon. Reviews help other readers discover this book and help me understand how the information resonated with you. Your feedback and insights mean so much, as they contribute to the ongoing development of resources like this, tailored for individuals who value fitness, peace, and independence.

Thank you once again, and here's to a lifetime of strength, health, and solo success!

-Jack

Resources:

1. Fitness Principles and Body Mechanics

- Books:
   - "Starting Strength: Basic Barbell Training" by Mark Rippetoe (2011).
   A comprehensive guide on strength training techniques and principles.

- "Strength Training Anatomy" by Frederic Delavier (2010).
   Illustrates the anatomy of strength training exercises, enhancing understanding of muscle engagement.

- Articles:
   - American Council on Exercise (ACE). "Muscle Fatigue vs. Muscle Soreness: What's the Difference?"
   Explains the physiological differences between muscle fatigue and soreness.
   [ACE Fitness Article](https://www.acefitness.org/education -and-resources/lifestyle/blog/6595/muscle-fatigue-vs-muscle -soreness-whats-the-difference/)

- National Institutes of Health (NIH). "The Importance of

Proper Form in Exercise."
Discusses the role of proper form in preventing injuries and maximizing workout effectiveness.
[NIH Article](https://www.ncbi.nlm.nih.gov/pmc/articles/PMC3371686/)

2. Goal Setting and Motivation

- Books:
  - "Atomic Habits: An Easy & Proven Way to Build Good Habits & Break Bad Ones" by James Clear (2018).
  Provides strategies for habit formation and goal setting.

- "Drive: The Surprising Truth About What Motivates Us" by Daniel H. Pink (2009).
  Explores intrinsic motivation and how it can be harnessed for personal growth.

- Articles:
  - Locke, E.A., & Latham, G.P. (2002). "Building a practically useful theory of goal setting and task motivation: A 35-year odyssey." American Psychologist, 57(9), 705-717.
  A seminal paper on goal-setting theory and its applications.

- MyFitnessPal. "The Benefits of Setting SMART Fitness Goals."
  Outlines the SMART framework for effective goal setting in fitness.
  [MyFitnessPal Article](https://blog.myfitnesspal.com/smart-goals-fitness/)

3. Tracking Progress and Celebrating Milestones

- Books:
   - "The Fitness Mindset: Eat for Energy, Train for Tension, Manage Your Mindset, Reap the Results" by Brian Keane (2017).
   Emphasizes the importance of tracking both physical and mental aspects of fitness.

- Articles:
   - Strava. "How to Track Your Fitness Progress Effectively."
   Provides tips on using fitness apps and trackers to monitor progress.
   [Strava Blog](https://blog.strava.com/how-to-track-your-fitness-progress-effectively/)

- Journal of Medical Internet Research (JMIR). "Effectiveness of Mobile Health Applications for Tracking Physical Activity and Fitness: A Systematic Review."
   Reviews the impact of mobile apps on fitness tracking and motivation.
   [JMIR Article](https://www.jmir.org/2020/4/e15866/)

4. Overcoming Plateaus and Introducing Variations

- Books:
   - "Bigger Leaner Stronger: The Simple Science of Building the Ultimate Male Body" by Michael Matthews (2012).
   Discusses strategies to overcome training plateaus and opti-

mize workouts.

- Articles:
  - Verywell Fit. "How to Overcome a Workout Plateau."
  Offers practical advice on breaking through fitness plateaus by varying workouts.
  [Verywell Fit Article](https://www.verywellfit.com/how-to-overcome-a-workout-plateau-1231206)

- National Strength and Conditioning Association (NSCA). "Progressive Overload: A Key to Successful Strength Training."
  Explains the principle of progressive overload and its role in continuous improvement.
  [NSCA Article](https://www.nsca.com/education/articles/most-exercise-scientists/progressive-overload-a-key-to-successful-strength-training/)

5. Mental Health and Mindfulness in Fitness

- Books:
  - "The Miracle of Mindfulness: An Introduction to the Practice of Meditation" by Thich Nhat Hanh (1975).
  Explores mindfulness practices that can be integrated into fitness routines.

- Articles:
  - Mayo Clinic. "Exercise and Stress: Get Moving to Manage Stress."
  Details the mental health benefits of regular exercise, includ-

ing stress reduction and improved mood.

[Mayo Clinic Article](https://www.mayoclinic.org/healthy-lifestyle/stress-management/in-depth/exercise-and-stress/art-20044469)

- Psychology Today. "Mindfulness and Fitness: How They Work Together."

Discusses the synergy between mindfulness practices and physical fitness.

[Psychology Today Article](https://www.psychologytoday.com/us/blog/the-athletes-way/201901/mindfulness-and-fitness-how-they-work-together)

6. Accountability and Support Systems

- Books:

- "The Power of Habit: Why We Do What We Do in Life and Business" by Charles Duhigg (2012).

Explores how habits are formed and the role of accountability in sustaining them.

- Articles:

- Harvard Business Review (HBR). "How Accountability Can Change Your Behavior."

Examines the psychological aspects of accountability and its impact on behavior change.

[HBR Article](https://hbr.org/2017/04/how-accountability-can-change-your-behavior)

- American Psychological Association (APA). "The Role of Accountability in Achieving Personal Goals."
Highlights the importance of accountability in personal goal attainment and provides strategies to enhance it.
[APA Article](https://www.apa.org/topics/accountability-personal-goals)

7. Nutrition and Recovery

- Books:
- "The New Rules of Lifting" by Lou Schuler and Alwyn Cosgrove (2010).
Covers comprehensive nutrition and recovery strategies to complement strength training.

- Articles:
- National Institutes of Health (NIH). "Nutrition and Physical Activity."
Provides guidelines on how proper nutrition supports physical activity and recovery.
[NIH Article](https://www.nutrition.gov/topics/basic-nutrition/physical-activity)

- PubMed Central (PMC). "The Role of Nutrition in Muscle Recovery and Growth."
Reviews the nutritional factors that aid in muscle recovery and growth post-exercise.
[PMC Article](https://www.ncbi.nlm.nih.gov/pmc/articles/PMC3905294/)

8. Flexibility and Mobility

- Books:
   - "Becoming a Supple Leopard" by Dr. Kelly Starrett (2013).
   A guide to improving mobility, flexibility, and overall movement quality.

- Articles:
   - Verywell Fit. "The Benefits of Flexibility Training."
   Explains how flexibility training enhances overall fitness and prevents injuries.
   [Verywell Fit Article](https://www.verywellfit.com/the-benefits-of-flexibility-training-1231244)

- National Academy of Sports Medicine (NASM). "The Importance of Flexibility in Fitness."
   Discusses the role of flexibility in maintaining a balanced fitness regimen.
   [NASM Article](https://www.nasm.org/blog/the-importance-of-flexibility-in-fitness)

9. Digital Tools and Technology in Fitness

- Books:
   - "Fitocracy: The Ultimate Book of Fitness Games and Challenges" by J.F. Dominguez (2013).
   Explores the use of gamification and technology in enhancing fitness motivation.

- Articles:
    - Journal of Medical Internet Research (JMIR). "Effectiveness of Mobile Health Applications for Tracking Physical Activity and Fitness: A Systematic Review."
    Analyzes the impact of mobile apps on fitness tracking and motivation.
    [JMIR Article](https://www.jmir.org/2020/4/e15866/)

- MyFitnessPal. "The Benefits of Using Fitness Apps for Tracking Progress."
    Details how fitness apps can aid in goal setting and progress monitoring.
    [MyFitnessPal Blog](https://blog.myfitnesspal.com/the-ben efits-of-using-fitness-apps-for-tracking-progress/)

10. Injury Prevention and Management

- Books:
    - "Overcoming Injury Through Sport Psychology" by John Bucher and Gavin Davidson (2005).
    Discusses psychological strategies for recovering from sports injuries.

- Articles:
    - American College of Sports Medicine (ACSM). "Injury Prevention and Safety."
    Provides guidelines on preventing injuries during exercise.
    [ACSM Article](https://www.acsm.org/read-research/resou rce-library/resource_detail?id=be0a7fda-6c91-4f9f-8e59-6e3

a2ff1d3d8)

- PubMed Central (PMC). "Preventing Injuries in Strength Training."
 Reviews strategies for minimizing the risk of injuries during strength training exercises.
 [PMC Article](https://www.ncbi.nlm.nih.gov/pmc/articles/PMC3761744/)

11. Mindfulness and Mental Health

- Books:
 - "Mindfulness for Beginners: Reclaiming the Present Moment—and Your Life" by Jon Kabat-Zinn (2015).
 Introduces mindfulness practices that can be integrated into fitness routines.

- Articles:
 - Psychology Today. "The Connection Between Mindfulness and Fitness."
 Explores how mindfulness enhances the effectiveness of physical workouts.
 [Psychology Today Article](https://www.psychologytoday.com/us/blog/the-athletes-way/201812/the-connection-between-mindfulness-and-fitness)

- Mayo Clinic. "Exercise and Stress: Get Moving to Manage Stress."
 Details the mental health benefits of regular exercise, includ-

ing stress reduction and improved mood.

[Mayo Clinic Article](https://www.mayoclinic.org/healthy-lifestyle/stress-management/in-depth/exercise-and-stress/art-20044469)

Supplementary Resources

- Websites:
  - American Council on Exercise (ACE): www.acefitness.org
  Offers a wealth of resources on exercise techniques, goal setting, and fitness education.

- National Strength and Conditioning Association (NSCA): www.nsca.com
  Provides research-based information on strength and conditioning.

- PubMed Central (PMC): www.ncbi.nlm.nih.gov/pmc/
  A free archive of biomedical and life sciences journal literature.

- Verywell Fit: www.verywellfit.com
  Features articles on fitness, nutrition, and wellness.

- Fitness Apps:
  - MyFitnessPal: [www.myfitnesspal.com](https://www.myfi

tnesspal.com)
   A comprehensive app for tracking diet and exercise.

- Strava: www.strava.com
   Popular among runners and cyclists for tracking workouts and connecting with a community.

- Fitbod: www.fitbod.me
   Generates personalized strength training workouts based on available equipment and goals.

9 798346 923497